Dialectic

Contributions to Human Development

Vol. 2

Series Editors
K. F. Riegel, Vancouver, B. C., and *H. Thomae,* Bonn

S. Karger · Basel · München · Paris · London · New York · Sydney

Dialectic

Humanistic Rationale for Behavior and Development

Volume Editor
J. F. Rychlak
Department of Psychological Sciences, Purdue University, West Lafayette, Ind.

S. Karger · Basel · München · Paris · London · New York · Sydney 1976

Contributions to Human Development
(Successor to 'Bibliotheca «Vita Humana»')

Vol. 1: *Thomae, H. and Endo, T.* (Bonn), ed.: The Adolescent and His Environment. Contributions to an Ecology of Teen-Age Behavior. VI + 110p., 6 fig., 6 tab., 1974. ISBN 3-8055-1651-7

Cataloging in Publication
Dialectic: humanistic rationale for behavior and development
Volume editor, J.F. Rychlak. Basel, New York, Karger, ©1976.
(Contributions to human development, v. 2)
1. Behavior 2. Psychological Theory
I. Rychlak, Joseph F., ed. II. Series
W1 C0778S v. 2/BF 204 D536
ISBN 3-8055-2288-6

Printed in Switzerland by Thür AG Offsetdruck, Pratteln
ISBN 3-8055-2288-6

Contents

Acknowledgment is made for permission to reprint the following materials:

Copyright 1956 by The David McKay Co., Inc. From the book *Taxonomy of Educational Objectives,* handbook I: The Cognitive Domain, edited by *B. S. Bloom.* Reprinted with permission of the publishers.

From *The Origins of Psycho-Analysis:* Letters to *Wilhelm Fliess,* Draft and Notes: 1887–1902, by *Sigmund Freud,* Edited by *Marie Bonaparte, Anna Freud, Ernst Kris,* Authorized Translation by *Eric Mosbacher* and *James Strachey,* (c) 1954 by Basic Books, Inc., Publishers, New York.

From *T. S. Kuhn, The Structure of Scientific Revolutions,* Second Edition, Copyright 1962, 1970, by the University of Chicago Press, Chicago.

From *Ulric Neisser, Cognitive Psychology,* Copyright 1967. Reprinted by permission of Prentice-Hall, Inc. Englewood Cliffs, N. J.

From *J. Piaget, Play, Dreams and Imitation in Childhood.* Copyright 1962. Reprinted by permission of W. W. Norton & Co., New York and Routledge & Kegan Paul, London.

Reprinted by permission of Yale University Press from *William Faulkner: The Yoknapatawpha Country* by Cleanth Brooks. Copyright (c) 1963 by Yale University.

Dedicated to the great dialecticians of history, including

Socrates	*Saint Augustine*	*Kierkegaard*
Mo Ti	*Maimonides*	*Marx*
Nāgārjuna	*Hegel*	*Freud*

Contributors to the Volume

Nancy Datan was born in Chicago, and took her MA and PhD degrees at the University of Chicago. A 10-year sojourn as a permanent resident of Israel separates her two graduate degrees; and in this interval her research as well as her experiences in transition between two cultures led to a commitment to the study of universally shaped and culturally mediated processes in personality development over the adult portion of the life cycle. She is presently a member of the Department of Psychology at West Virginia University.

Robert Hogan was born in Los Angeles, attended the University of California at Los Angeles, and took his PhD at the University of California at Berkeley. He is interested in personality theory, personality assessment, and moral development. He is currently on the faculty of Psychology at The Johns Hopkins University.

Steinar Kvale is Norwegian. He took the doctoral degree at the University of Oslo, and is presently teaching at the University of Aarhus in Denmark. Dr. *Kvale* was a research Scholar at the University of Heidelberg and he has been a visiting professor at Duquesne University. He has published works on memory and examinations, reflecting a phenomenological and dialectical approach to psychology.

Susan V. Lourenço was born in England and obtained MA degrees at both Oxford and Columbia Universities before taking the doctoral degree at the University of Chicago. She was a Program Director with the Center for the Teaching Professions, Northwestern University, as well as an Assistant Professor in the School of Education. Dr. *Lourenço* has considerable experience as an educator and researcher. She is now an Associate Professor of Psychology in the European Division of George Peabody's Overseas Human Development Counseling Program. Her published work reflects the themes of social dynamics, conflict, values, and the educational process.

James C. Mancuso followed a standard educational program to complete his PhD at the University of Rochester, N. Y. Five years of effort to use psychological formulations in applied settings convinced him that psychologists first need to evolve a cohesive view of persons, and he therefore assumed an academic career at the State University of New York at Albany. In his position as Professor of Psychology he explores personality theories and investigates problems related to the development of person-construing processes.

Klaus F. Riegel obtained his doctoral degree at the University of Hamburg and has been in the United States since that time, first at the National Institute of Mental Health, Bethesda, and then at the University of Michigan. Dr. *Riegel* is known for his work in psychological gerontology and developmental psychology with an emphasis on language and cognition. During recent years he has revived his long-term interest in theoretical and historical studies of individual and social changes.

Joseph F. Rychlak took the doctoral degree at The Ohio State University and is now Professor of Psychology at Purdue University. Trained as a clinical psychologist and psychotherapist, Dr. *Rychlak* gradually moved to an interest in the basic learning principles involved in human behavior. His Logical Learning Theory has been framed as a humanistic alternative to the prevalent mechanistic learning theories of modern psychology.

Robert J. Sardello received his BA degree from St. Mary's University in San Antonio, Tex., and his MS and PhD in Experimental Psychology from Saint Louis University. At present he is Chairman of the Department of Psychology and Director of the Graduate Program of Psychology in the Institute of Philosophic Studies at the University of Dallas. He has written in the areas of human learning and cognitive development, imagination, fantasy, memory, laughter, myth, and hermeneutics. His current work centers on a psychological hermeneutics of classical mythology, relating this work to the tradition of depth psychology.

Kuo You-yuh, born and reared in China, earned his doctoral degree at the University of Maryland. Now on the faculty of Psychology at Ball State University, he has published articles in American and Chinese journals on the themes of educational philosophy, juvenile delinquency, and creativity. He is also interested in a dialectical theory of motivation and in translating learning principles and theories into practical teaching strategies for developing intellectual abilities.

Addresses of the Contributors

Nancy Datan, PhD, Department of Psychology, West Virginia University, Morgantown, WV 26506 (USA)

Robert Hogan, PhD, Department of Psychology, The Johns Hopkins University, Baltimore, MD 21218 (USA)

Steinar Kvale, PhD, Institute of Psychology, University of Aarhus, 4 Asylvej, 8240 Risskov, Denmark

You-Yuh Kuo, Ed. D., Department of Educational Psychology, Ball State University, Muncie, IN 47306 (USA)

Susan V. Lourenço, PhD, George Peabody College for Teachers, Program in Human Development Counseling, Peabody Regional Center, APO, NY 09194 (USA)

James Mancuso, PhD, Department of Psychology, State University of New York at Albany, 1400 Washington Avenue, Albany, NY 12203 (USA)

Klaus F. Riegel, PhD, Department of Psychology, The University of British Columbia, Vancouver V6T 1W5 (Canada)

Joseph F. Rychlak, PhD, Dept. of Psychological Sciences, Purdue University, West Lafayette, IN 47907 (USA)

Robert J. Sardello, PhD, Department of Psychology, University of Dallas, Irving, TX 75060 (USA)

Introduction

This book has one unifying theme, which frames its purpose and invites the reader to challenge his or her thinking concerning just what a science of humanity should have to account for. We are trying to publicize the currently underestimated and often misunderstood concept of dialectic in psychological theorizing. Although it is not essential for dialectical theories to be humanisms, it is my personal belief that there are several compelling reasons for describing human behavior less mechanistically if we but acknowledge the dialectical side to it. No properly educated social scientist today should presume to speak for the behavior of human beings without a good understanding of the dialectical metaconstruct. Yet few modern psychological theorists seem aware of its existence in the history of thought, much less employ its heuristic benefits in their formal views. So, there is much work to be done by those of us who find this side to the human image essential. The hope is that this volume as a first effort will lay down a general direction which others can follow who see the necessity of dealing with *all* aspects of human behavior and development.

Five of the chapters in this volume were delivered as papers at the 80th Annual Convention of the American Psychological Association (Honolulu, Hawaii, September 1972). Two of the chapters have appeared in print before, although they have been edited considerably, and one of these was written initially for this volume. Six chapters are entirely new writings, neither appearing in print before nor having been delivered as talks. The writing and editing has proven to be a pleasant experience, with the contributors marvelously helpful and even dedicated to their task. The pleasure and ease of this work was undoubtedly due to the fact that my wife, *Lenora*, took on much of the editorial responsibility. I would sincerely like to thank her for her efforts.

Joseph F. Rychlak

Contr. hum. Dev., vol. 2, pp. 1–17 (Karger, Basel 1976)

Chapter 1
The Multiple Meanings of 'Dialectic'

Joseph F. Rychlak

Though the social sciences began to emerge before its turn, surely the 20th Century has been of extreme importance to the growth of psychology, sociology, political science, and so forth. If the 17th Century provided the philosophical-theoretical rationale for a natural science, then the century in which we now live is equally pertinent to the acceptable conceptualizations of a science of human behavior and social institutions. The leading 17th Century thinkers – *Bacon, Descartes, Galileo, Hobbes, Locke, Leibniz, Newton*, etc. – were cognizant of the demands put on them as trailblazers in science. This prompted them to consider the various practices of their speciality, its assumptions, prescriptions, and the directions it ought to take. It seems to be tacitly accepted by all today that these 17th Century prescriptions and recommended procedures are 'given' for all time, and that any reexamination of our major heuristic schemes can only be prompted by a nonscientific or antiscientific motivation.

This attitude is not only incorrect but highly injurious since it negates rigorous thinking and self-criticism among those scientists who need such self-examination the most. We refer here to the social scientists who have so readily patterned their conceptual models on the paradigms of natural science (*Kuhn*, 1970). It is the purpose of the present volume to show how this naive acceptance of natural-science description has eclipsed a vital side of human nature, one which *must* be captured if social science is ever to achieve credibility. This side has to do with the *dialectic* or *dialectical* description of behaviors, events, societies, and so on. Here is an ancient conception so pervasive in human affairs, so pregnant with meaning for analysis, so useful as heuristic aid that to have ignored it these many decades into the 20th Century almost constitutes an act of irresponsibility on the part of 'modern' social science. We hope to rectify this oversight in the present volume.

Outside of the Communist orbit, the only scholarly work on the dialectic in this century was done by *Adler*, whose book *Dialectic* (1927) and treatment of the topic in the *Syntopicon* (1952) of the *Great Books of the Western World* series are excellent sources for study. What one immediately discovers in such study is that there is no single view of dialectic to 'define' as representative of the conception for all time. The concept is as elusive as the human beings who behave according to its descriptive characterizations, or employ it to make sense out of some topic of their interest. Indeed, the elusive definitional quality of the dialectic merely reflects a central characteristic of the conception *per se.* Dialectical formulations are ever restless, on the move, and unwilling to be pinned down for any length of time. To freeze dialectic into a single, fixed definition would be to destroy it. Once the reader accepts this fluid idea of dialectical change and development, a host of life experiences will be seen to fall within its range of descriptive convenience. Moreover, the conceptualizations of behavior which result will invariably be *more human.* As the title of our volume suggests, the dialectic always serves as the rationale for a humanistic science – almost 'by definition'. That is, dialectical formulations are anathema to mechanistic accounts, and psychology to this point in time has most surely been a predominantly mechanistic science.

What, then, can anyone mean by 'dialectic'? In this chapter we will review several ways in which the concept has been employed by thinkers across the ages. Without trying to fix a single definition we will prepare the reader for the chapters to follow, in which a series of psychologists with different specialties and different commitments to the dialectical construct will be seen to put their ideas to work.

Dialectic as a World Principle

One of the oldest manifestations of dialectical theorizing is to be found in its use as a 'world principle'. In the very first *recorded* philosophical treatise of Western thought, *Anaximander* (c.611–547 BC) of Miletus argued that the elements of the universe were held together by an opposition – air is cold, fire is hot, and so forth. *Heraclitus* (540–480 BC) was later to say that *strife* is the principle of change by which events moved across time. This emanated from the fact that opposition was fundamental to all life; even so, said *Heraclitus*, the opposite poles of a bipolarity in meaning are 'the same' (so that, e. g., left means right). *Empedocles* (493–433 BC) next held that 'love and strife' were the dialectical antagonists which moved events. In the philosophy of *Socrates* (470–399 BC) and *Plato* (427–346 BC), the movement from the world of everyday events (Becoming) to the realm of pure ideas (Being) was made possible thanks to the fact that all meanings were tied together dialectically into a totality of seemingly unrelated significations (*Plato*, 1952). We shall return to this point in the next section. Historians have long noted that the Graecian mind was a universal mind thanks to the fact that it viewed all things in nature as dialectically related. Hence, knowledge, understanding, intellectual perspective was 'all of one piece' (*Becker and Barnes*, 1952).

We should not be misled into believing that dialectical formulations were limited to Western thought. The role of Buddhism in shaping Eastern thought is often stressed by scholars, who characterize the peculiarities of Indian, Chinese, and Japanese thought by the ways in which these peoples have assimilated Buddhistic concepts (see, e. g., *Nākāmura*, 1964). And Buddhism is a heavily dialectical view of life in the universe. The predominant theme running through both the Hindu and Buddhistic philosophies of India is the necessary search for a oneness in nature, the breaking down of false dichotomies, and a unity in the totality of experience which results in 'liberation' *(moksa)* or 'nirvana' (*Moore*, 1967 b). Turning to Chinese thought, the renowned text, the *Tao Te Ching* (c. 600 BC, probably of multiple authorship) is replete with dialectical conceptions, the most famous of which is the *yin* and *yang* principle. The *yin* force or element is pictured as passive, receiving, and meek (on the face of things); yet, like the female or mother, *yin* represents the potential for infinite creation in the world. The *yang* force is more active and bold, reflecting its power overtly in a more masculine sense. Harmony as a kind of dialectical balance between *yin* and *yang* is most desirable, although it is also true that the Chinese character prefers to display its *yin* side and keep *yang* inclinations in the background (*Moore*, 1967 a). In Chapter 8 we shall have a more detailed presentation of the *yin-yang* principle, especially as background to the dialectical interpretations of *Mao Tse-tung*, which takes us to our next example under the present heading.

Doubtless the most important dialectical world principle of our time is the Marxian (*Marx*, 1952) formulation, which is a materialistic re-casting of the Hegelian conception of God, coming to consciousness by way of dialectical movements across history. This development took the form of repeated *theses, antitheses* and *syntheses* (*Hegel*, 1952, p. 53; *Hook*, 1962 p. 54). Whereas *Hegel* (1770–1831) spoke of the contradictions in the 'spirits' of peoples which clashed and changed across the ages, *Marx* (1818–1883) put this opposition in economic forces and the resultant class struggle. The dialectical march across history was inexorable, and the outcome certain. God would achieve self-consciousness and the final 'negation of a negation' in the progression of *dialectical materialism* would end in the classless state. *Marx* observed that the dialectic in material nature was 'a scandal and an abomination to bourgeoisdom and its doctrinaire professors because it includes in its comprehension an affirmative recognition of the existing state of things, [and] at the same time, also, the recognition of the negation of that state, of its inevitable breaking up . . .' (*Marx*, 1952, p. 11).

This threatening sense of confidence in the inevitable collapse of capitalism is at least one of the reasons for the unpopularity of dialectical conceptions today. There are many people who naively assume that 'dialectic' means *only* 'dialectical materialism' in the history of thought. The truth is, there are dialecticians in history who would contend that one *cannot* predict the inexorable course of a dialectical conception (see Chapter 12 on this point). In a dialectical confrontation or contradiction, if the outcome is known beforehand then a truly dialectical encounter would not have taken place. As we shall see in the next section, this is how *Socrates* viewed the dialectic conception. Furthermore, by ending their dialectic in a specific social order, both *Hegel* and *Marx* effectively destroyed the likelihood of dialectical advance from that point onward.

Dialectic as Valid Organon

The next meaning of dialectic we might single out has to do with its use as a valid organon – i. e., as a correct means or manner for coming to know truth. When we deal with knowledge we invariably commit ourselves to the question of *meaning*. The word 'meaning' has Anglo-Saxon roots in 'to wish' and 'to intend', which immediately suggests a directional pointing or inferential suggestion, whereby some 'given' heralds 'something else'. Whether we consider a word or an image, the suggestion in 'meaning' is that there is a relational tie of 'this' item with one or more 'other' items, patterning the several items into a totality. But the basic pattern here, the most simple pattern possible, seems to be a bipolarity. Dialecticians have always insisted that meanings *are* bipolar in this fashion. Even the seeming unipolar act of pointing to some object which one 'means' to bring to someone's attention is seen as a bipolar act of suggesting 'that is that' or 'that is what you should be aware of'. Of course, some dialecticians would say that there is no need to presume *all* meanings to be bipolar, just so we appreciate that many are. In addition to suggesting that we could not know 'left' without knowing 'right' (refer above), *Heraclitus* used a dialectical rationale when he said that we could not appreciate acts of justice if it were not for acts of injustice in human affairs. The 'negative' side of behavior helps mankind appreciate the positive.

There are decided implications here for conceptions of morality and ethics in human relations. Dialectical formulations lend themselves to theories of morality and ethics, and we shall see this application of a dialectical theory in Chapter 6. Theologians have often employed dialectical theories to make their case. For example, the concept of 'negative theology', as practiced in the Hebrew faith by *Maimonides* (1135–1204) and in the Catholic faith by *Saint Bonaventura* (1221–1274), is an example of a dialectical organon. Because God is such an inscrutable and awe-inspiring conception, it is fitting that we admit ignorance in affirmative terms. As creatures far below this ascendant meaning, we move from the unipolar 'is' to its opposite, and attempt to say what God *is not*.

Theologians frequently rely on dialectical formulations as a kind of 'personal organon' through which the individual has the capacity of opting for the 'good' (God's will) in life. Since good and evil are dialectical opposites, the direction actually taken in behavior is to some extent 'up to the person'. Modern psychology has no inkling of this dialectical conception, since it views behavior in quite other terms – terms we shall consider in the next section. But whether they are aware of it or not, theologians have for centuries relied upon dialectical logic to explain 'free will'. In the more distant past, *Origen*'s (c.185–c.254) concept of the Fall of Divine Powers was of this sort. The Good – as created by God – would have no meaning without its opposite Evil as a potentiality in even Divine Affairs. Quite clearly, an option for Evil *had* to exist since it was pointless to speak of Good otherwise. Hence, it was simply a question of time before the opposite possibility was affirmed by Divinities which had this option open to them as dialectical beings. Centuries later, *Kierkegaard* (1813–1855) was to root his existentialistic philosophy and capacity for an 'either/or' decision on precisely this kind of 'subjective dialectic' in the functioning of human beings. That is, *Kierkegaard* took his dialectic out of the World Principle (Hegelian) type of formulation and put it subjectively in the breast of every human being who must now opt and commit himself to some course of action since that is the nature of life.

In Oriental philosophy, a school of dialectical thought also evolved, stemming in large measure from the writings of *Mo Ti* (c.470–c.391 BC) who said that the dialectic was a method to be used in identifying right from wrong, good from bad, and similarity from difference. *Kun-sun Lung* (c.330–250 BC) subsequently noted that all things are but a manifestation of unchanging universals, made clear to man's senses by oppositional ties in the concrete particulars of everyday events. This philosophy is remarkably like the Socratic-Platonic distinction between the realm of Being (unchanging universals) and the realm of Becoming (concrete particulars in which universals participate), to which we now turn.

If the average person does not immediately think of 'dialectical materialism' when the term 'dialectic' is dropped into the conversation, then he most surely thinks of a 'questions and answers' procedure employed by *Socrates* in his unique style of instruction and/or search for knowledge. The 'dialogues' (*Plato*, 1952) present us with this procedure, in which *Socrates* would pose a question for his student to take a stand on, and then defend the point in opposition to the student's. If the student chose A, *Socrates* defended not-A; if the student chose not-A, *Socrates* defended A. It was all the same to him, for *Socrates* did not think of himself as having 'knowledge' stored within a memory bank to 'communicate' from his head to the student's head. Whatever he knew as an individual, the other person being questioned *also* knew. Working together, dialectically examining the potential knowledge *both* persons in the dialogue possessed, two people could learn purely through verbal examination. Beginning in admitted error, they could come to know its opposite – truth! – because all things are united through such opposition (refer above).

Since *Plato* recorded these discussions as an unfolding exchange between student and teacher, it sometimes appears to the reader that *Socrates* was cleverly and subtly directing the conversation to a predetermined end. It is as if the dialogue followed a scenario. But this was precisely what *Socrates* was trying to avoid! His intention was to keep the conversation open, free to move in *any* direction imaginable, depending only on what would emerge in the free exchange of ideas. If a person employed dialectical questioning techniques in order to direct a conversation or course of verbal investigation to some predetermined end, *Socrates* would have called this *sophistry* (i. e., an insincere, often specious, but deceptively subtle line of argumentation). This is what the Greek Sophists did and *Socrates* took great delight in tripping up these superficial debators and teachers. The spirit of dialectical discourse in the Socratic sense is ever-open to the spontaneous possibilities in things. Anything suggested in the exchange is to be given legitimate consideration, for both sides are open to discovery as neither can know where the verbal exchange will end. Indeed, the dialectical process of discovery is never ending. The questions raised by dialectical examination often exceed those which are answered. 'Final answers' are not always forthcoming in any case. The certainty which *Marx* assigned to the march of dialectic in material reality is thus not to be seen in the intellectual interpretation of dialectic profferred by *Socrates* (refer above).

Dialectic as Invalid Organon

Sophistry brings us to another view of the dialectic, and that is as *invalid* organon promoting mistakes in logic *whenever it is employed*. In other words, there can be no possible use for dialectic at all because it is literally the father of error. A heuristic procedure which views error as a 'something', as an active principle in the generation of knowledge, results in quite different forms of understanding than a procedure which presumes that error is a 'nothing', an irrelevant state of affairs in relation to what is the truth. It was *Aristotle* who altered the view of error in our intellectual heritage, even as he introduced a style of thought aimed at rigorously removing – or at least limiting – man's reliance upon dialectical logic. *Aristotle* (1952) rankled at the 'armchair' features of the Socratic dialectic, where two men talked and talked, often fooling themselves into believing that they were coming to know truth when in fact they were simply perpetuating error by way of personal opinions. *Aristotle* formulated the first clearly 'toughminded' philosophy when he denied that one can begin in *error* and come to know truth. Unfounded premises can only lead to unfounded conclusions. *Aristotle* did not deny that man *could* reason dialectically. He acknowledged that when under attack concerning our major premises we all must resort to a dialectical defense – since often there is no real 'proof' that one premise is any more valid than another. In a situation of this type we all become sophists. But, this is no reason to court sophistry as a primary or 'scientific' organon.

What *Aristotle* was to accomplish in his critique was to shift man's attention to the extraction (usually called 'deduction') of knowledge from premises, whereas dialecticians had always been more interested in the *framing* of these premises (usually called 'induction'). The dialectician is a seeker, and he appreciates his unique role in the actual creation of knowledge. We find dialecticians emphasizing the questions of how we interpret events, our points of view, the contradictions in seemingly pat events depending upon the 'slant' we take in construing them, and so forth. *Marx*, for example, insisted that historical events were not simply 'there' for understanding but had to be interpreted – and one's interpretation depended on his class identity which *had* to exert an influence. Living within an historical period, one might be so caught up in the sway of events that he is incapable of knowing what forces are at play. Subsequently, however, a proper dialectical examination will enlighten the historian who must perforce apply his frame of reference to events in *post hoc* fashion. In this case we speak of the single human being as reflecting a class bias, but a directly comparable view of dialectical examination can be seen in *Kierkegaard*'s belief that the individual must commit himself to his subjectively arrived at (via dialectical examination) 'position' on a life event and thence to 'act' according to his commitment. Whether personal behavior or one's interpretation of history, the dialectical framing of events puts the human person at the forefront in the *creation* (induction, construing, premising) of knowledge.

Aristotle, on the other hand, focuses primarily on the *extraction* of knowledge from premises already framed! He drew a distinction between two forms of reasoning or logical progressions (Organons); one was a *demonstrative* progression and the other a *dialectical*. The heart of this distinction has to do with how we arrive at our (especially 'major') premises preliminary to extracting (deducting) the meanings implied therein. Whereas dialecticians base their premises on mere *opinion* – as when *Socrates* initiated a dialogue by putting some question like 'What is Beauty? ' to a student who then answered with his view – the demonstrative reasoner relies on only *primary and true* meanings to initiate and thereby guide a course of thought. *Aristotle* had various rules for what a primary and true premise was, but the essential notion here was of a *unipolarity* in meaningful denotation. One cannot take an 'either-or' stance on the truth-value of a primary and true premise.

For example, the tautology 'All bachelors are unmarried males' is unipolar and not open to the challenge of a contrary opinion. Another primary and true premise would be any empirical 'fact', as an operational definition of what is truly the case in reality. *Aristotle* was the father of biology precisely because he wished to turn our attention away from exclusive reliance on dialectical discussion to the empirically discernible facts of existence. An operational definition is actually a variant tautology, as when we say 'That measure (X) is my concept (X), for the purpose of this study.' We do not always appreciate the 'That is that' or 'X is X' feature of such statements, but they all come down to an effort to turn a bipolarity into a unipolarity in meaningful designation. There can be no nonsense about what is affirmed, no dialectical tricks or sophistical twists in the meaning to be extracted from such 'givens'. Some dialecticians would insist that even a tautology is bipolar, but others would agree that in this case the two ends of a 'that is that' statement reflect a unipolarity (see our discussion of meaning in the previous section).

This distinction between dialectical and demonstrative reasoning strategies can be shown to permeate the theologies and philosophies which have emerged down through history. In theology, for example, *Saint Augustine* (354–430) was a complete dialectician, whose Holy Trinity conception is but one manifestation of this proclivity to see events complexly. *Saint Thomas Aquinas* (1225–1274) was closer to *Aristotle* in his suspicion over the possible misuse of dialectical reasoning – though he never denied that man could, after all, 'reason by opposites'. *William of Ockham* (c.1280–c.1350), on the other hand, essentially reified *Aristotle*'s demonstrative reasoning conception into a physical model of man. That is, he distinguished between knowing things intuitively via sensory input, and knowing things abstractly, based on 'merely' mental ratiocinations after sensory input had taken place (*Magill* and *McGreal*, 1961, p. 337). Since knowledge or 'information', as we call it today, was brought into mind via the senses and since the senses were *unidirectional* and *unipolar* in their structure (nerves send 'a' signal, not 'two or more' signals), the upshot is that knowledge was said to *always* begin in empirical reality. Knowledge was 'out there', and then brought 'in here', to work mentally in what is effectively a demonstrative form of thought-making. That is, dialectical reasoning was now relegated to some kind of *erroneous* processing of input information. Dialectical reasoning was always specious, nothing but error, hence it was to that extent *nothing*!

It is this complete dismissal of dialectical reasoning in the human image which we see arising in the philosophy of British Empiricism, aided and abetted by the parallel rise in mathematics over the 16th and 17th centuries. Mathematical reasoning is surely the *sine qua non* of demonstrative reasoning, in which *Aristotle*'s 'law of contradiction' holds without question – i. e., 'A is not not-A'. This is flatly nondialectical, of course, for dialecticians view even contradictory statements or paradoxes as potentially holding the greatest kinds of truth. We find the British Empiricists effectively mathematizing the concept of mind. *Hob-*

bes (1588–1679; 1952) was fond of saying that 'Thinking is reckoning [i. e., adding and subtracting]' and *Locke* (1632–1704; 1952) drew many parallels to mathematics as he turned man's reason into a 'probability estimate' for today based upon the frequency of this or that kind of sensory input from out of the past (*Ockham*'s intuitive cognition). Dialectical reasoning fell completely from this account, and since it is the Lockean model which functions today as the unquestioned institutionalized paradigm of academic psychology, it is impossible to find a current theoretical account in which humans might be said to 'reason by opposites'. Thanks to the rise of natural science, a demonstrative strategy in rigorous experimentation has served the ancillary role of eclipsing dialectic as a possible model for human behavior. The logic runs something like this: Dialectical formulations embrace error. Psychology is a science and is therefore opposed to error. Conclusion? Dialectical theories are unamenable to a science of psychology. Sound enough, so far as it goes. But what if humans *do* reason dialectically?

There is a parallel development of the dialectical versus demonstrative variety in Oriental philosophy. We have already identified the Dialectical School of *Mo Ti* and *Kung-sun Lung*, above. *Confucius* (c.551–c.479 BC), on the other hand, propounded a school of thought which was lacking in dialectical formulations (*Magill and McGreal*, 1961; *Moore*, 1967 a). As with the clarity emphasis of a demonstrative logic, Confucian philosophy called for a distinctly ordered, harmonious and regularized society without strife and deferent to tradition. Propriety defines a unipolarity, since it is presumed that there *is* a right and a wrong way to behave. Hence, 'pure' Confucianism is nondialectical though, in the course of time, Confucian themes were combined with yin-yang principles and a form of Neo-Confucianism arose which was to predominate in prerevolutionary China (see Chapter 8).

Dialectic as Transcendence

The Ockham-Hobbes-Locke line of argument, which held that 'information' was brought into the mind as input influences, to be combined into various probable output occurrences based on their frequency distributions gives us a thoroughly mechanistic interpretation of intelligence. This style of reasoning is best exemplified in the thinking of a cybernetics machine. Propositions fed into the machine are either true or false, and in no case is something both true *and* false (law of contradiction). If an error is discerned, this is tantamount to saying 'truth' has not developed, so the machine simply stops functioning because it is not equipped to deal with 'error'. The oft-cited fact that thinking machines do not make mistakes is simply the other side of the fact that they cannot create anything. They are like demonstrative creatures who can only extract or deduct information from the *unquestioned* meanings as framed in the primary and true premises which are fed to them. It is the operator of the machine who puts these premises into the machine that must face the possibility of error.

But what are we now to say when modern learning theories attempt to describe the human operator in precisely identical terms? If, as we contend, the institutionalized paradigm of psychology is Lockean (*Kuhn*, 1970), how can the human being operating the thinking machine be said to differ from it in any significant extent? He cannot, of course, and therefore it is not surprising to find that psychology has effectively foreclosed on a dialectical image of man. Human behavior (as all behavior) is conceptualized as an unidirectional input-output succession of events, with various mediators functioning as probabilistic 'determiners' of action (*Rychlak*, 1968, pp. 362–366). Mediators are past inputs, etched onto the *tabula rasa* mind *(Locke)* by the intuitive cognition *(Ockham)* after birth and functioning according to a mathematical principle of frequency and contiguity in subsequent time. Errors reduce themselves to inadequate or erroneous inputs, incorrect encodings of such inputs, loss at the level of storage, inability to reclaim stored information (memory) due to interference, and so forth. Mind (as all events) flows along in that substrate reality of efficient causation which natural science has presumed *can only* develop in a unidirectional, demonstrative manner.

Straining against this British Empiricistic conception of mind, however, we find the more Continental line of philosophy as epitomized by *Kant* (1724–1804). Though *Kant* was just as wary of the free play of dialectical speculation as were *Aristotle* and *Aquinas* before him, he appreciated as they had that human reason *did* function by way of bipolarity and opposition in meaning-enlargement. *Ockham* had made intuitive cognition seem a completely unstructured occurrence, in the sense of what the individual *qua* person did to the input of sensory experience. Actually, *Kant* argued, sensory input is always organized by the person in terms of both space and time. Space and time factors are not 'in' the sensory input, but are placed onto them by the phenomenal grasp of experience which each person brings to raw experience. This capacity for mental organization is even more important in reasoning, because when we speculate in pure reason it is possible to have ideas which *transcend* sensory experience (intuitive cognition) entirely (*Kant*, 1952, p. 115). Knowledge can begin in experience, as organized by sensory factors, but it does not always arise out of experience *as input*, because in pure reason – i. e., free thought – it is possible to have ideas which are totally unrelated to 'external reality'.

This can occur because of the functioning in mind of a *transcendental dialectic* permitting us to concoct fanciful and highly distorted versions of that which we perceive daily through reasoning by opposites, and opposites of opposites, until we have removed ourselves from the realm of familiar events and known 'facts'. Mind will have created something completely outside of and beyond experience – an in that magnificient, substantial example of the Sphinx which has a human head and an animal body. What thinking machine could have concocted such an *untrue* possibility from out of its electrically mediated inputs? Yet, there it stands, a monument to the dialectical intelligence of human beings. Had Moses fed his program of Ten Commandments into a newly created crop of cybernetic-beings, we never would have had the Fall of Divine Powers which *Origen* accounted for dialectically (refer above). An exclusively demonstrative human being could never see the immediate lascivious possibilities in the supposedly unipolar designation of 'Thou shalt not covet thy neighbor's wife'.

The philosophies of the East were also infused with dialectical transcendentalism (*Moore*, 1967 b). The Indian Buddhist *Nāgārjuna* (c.100–150 AD) denied or negated the world of phenomenal experience through four paired oppositions: i. e., neither birth nor death, neither permanence nor extinction, neither unity nor diversity, and neither coming nor going (*Moore*, 1967 b, p. 112). We have here a form of the 'negation of a negation' theme mentioned above as typical of Hegelian and Marxian formulations, except that *Nāgārjuna* was saying that the Buddhistic Monk could reach the Middle Path *(nirvāṅa)* only by transcending the oppositional tensions of existence and moving toward Emptiness *(sunyata)* and Void *(sunya)*. Zen Buddhism has a comparable emphasis, in which Perfect Enlightenment is achieved only after the student transcends his question-answer, true-false, law-of-contradiction approach to knowledge and achieves a higher state of 'oneness' with the Universe. This takes us into the final interpretation which dialectic is likely to be given.

Dialectic as Many in One

The final meaning of dialectic we would like to draw the reader's attention to is already implied in the meanings surveyed above. It is in many ways the most important usage for psychology, and can be seen as a principle in opposition to the so-called law of contradiction. Since the earliest days of philosophical discourse it has been mentioned as the 'many in one' or 'one in many' thesis – with variations stated as one and many, many among one, and so forth. This assumption of a unity within diversity is what provided the Greek dialecticians with their world view enabling discriminations to be made via a dialectical organon. How one slices up this pie of 'totality' is basically arbitrary, since through dialectical examination it can always be shown how 'this difference' between A and not-A is really a form of 'identity' when looked at via the perspectives of X, Y, and Z. To hold that a thing cannot both be and not be at the same time is just not true, to a dialectician. *Hegel* once framed an argument proving that a thing could both be and not be at the same time (*Stace*, 1955, p. 90). *Saint Augustine*'s Holy Trinity conception, which we mentioned above, is another example of the same identity being both more and less than what it is depending upon just how one looks at the totality.

Now, of course, the immediate rejoinder to this kind of talk by a person falling back on demonstrative tactics is that such arguments or conceptions are all nonsense. Dialectical machinations of this sort perpetuate error and mistakes. They cannot be taken seriously. If we view this situation from the point of view of methodological validation, we are forced to admit that the demonstratively reasoning critic has a good point to make. It would simply not do to have a scientific method in which left could mean right, up could mean down, and findings in one direction could mean their opposite. The writer has argued that this is precisely what happened in the evolution of psychoanalysis, which is an expressed effort at science that made use of dialectical formulations as *proof* (*Rychlak*, 1973, p. 227). In his 1908 correspondence with *Jung*, *Freud* tells of a principle of proof he has worked out with *Ferenczi* to the effect: 'What paranoiacs tell us is false; i. e., the opposite is true' (*McGuire*, 1974, p. 191). *Freud* actually held to this kind of view for all of his patients when the material being denied was given particular emphasis (see, e. g., *Freud*, 1961, p. 235). To negate something vehemently is to essentially say 'I would rather repress this than have to deal with it.'

Though this might be true for paranoiacs or psychoanalytical patients, it is hardly a principle on the basis of which we can found a science. Insights such as these can even be studied by way of translating the theoretical formulation into variables in experimental design and predicting to a certain outcome accordingly ('control and prediction' in the process of validating evidence; see *Rychlak*, 1968, p. 77). But to make dialectic into a method of proof *per se* is surely risky business, considering the potentials it has for sophistical and erroneous commentary. On the other hand, it is equally risky business to go on denying the theoretical possibility of dialectical reasoning in human behavior. If *Freud* has regrettably forced his dialectical theory of human behavior onto the methods of science, then the reverse is surely true of modern experimental psychology. As we have seen above, modern psychology has pressed its demonstrative style of reasoning in its approach to proof onto its very conception of behavior. It has done what *Burtt* (1955, p. 229) said Newtonian Science had done earlier, and that is to make a metaphysics out of its method.

It is important to take up the question of proof in a book on the dialectic, because no one should be misled into thinking that a dialectician cannot have the utmost regard for scientific rigor. We shall even have examples in the present volume (see especially Chapters 6, 7, 9, 10, and 11) in which empirical efforts are made to scientifically validate (method) conceptions (theories) based on a dialectical formulation. Our real problem at this point in history is to convince social scientists that something like the dialectic might really be going on in this world of interpersonal, social, and historical forces. Once this premise is entertained, once this 'paradigm' is accepted as worthy of application, then as *Kuhn* (1970, pp. 23–42) has taught us in his conception of 'normal science', it will be possible to do empirical studies in rigorous support of this conception. As of now there is no way of proving that which effectively is said *not* to exist!

It was probably the gestalt psychologists more than any other who popularized this meaning in their claim that the 'whole is more than simply the sum of its parts'. *Koffka* (1886–1941; 1935) lamented the endless round of reductions which Lockean theorists seemed to demand in coming to their scientific explanations. This reductive orientation, contended *Koffka* (1935, p. 9), arbitrarily chose to ignore many aspects of man's existence; it was his hope in time to alter the approach to science in psychology and thereby help 'recreate that original unity which it had to destroy in order to develop'. Of course, this did not mean that the gestaltists made use of a dialectical conception in accounting for their theories of behavior. The gestaltists were children of their time and therefore did not embrace a concept of transcendental dialectic in their otherwise very Kantian theories of perception and thinking. Such 'unpredictable' conceptions were no more welcome in their camp than they were in the Lockean camps of the time.

An even clearer source of one-in-many theories has been the psychiatric or psychological consulting room. As already implied in our comments on *Freud* above, the writings of the psychoanalysts and later personality-psychotherapists who followed in their wake are often fraught with unnamed dialectical theories of behavior – masked under the designations of irony, paradox, self-destructiveness, 'insane logic', and the like. Chapter 4 will take up this very important application of dialectical theory, so we shall forego a more detailed commentary in the present chapter. There are also clearly dialectical theories alive in theories of aesthetics and artistic expression. Typically, one finds that artistic expression, to be accurately grasped, demands a 'tension of opposites' phrasing in which the totality subsumes some such internal counterplay of aesthetic effects. In his four-volume work, *The Social History of Art*, *Hauser* uses this device in discussing architecture (1951, vol. I, p. 242), the drama (vol. III, p. 85), the novel (vol. IV, p. 28), and painting (vol. IV, p. 168). Each art form is seen to lend itself to a dialectical analysis. Music has been said to be a highly versatile art form because it permits the simultaneous expression of opposite tones and emotionally expressive melodies (*Langer*, 1948, p. 48). Yet, psychology has not seen fit to apply a dialectical model to its aesthetic theories. In Chapters 2 and 3 we shall see a beginning effort to deal with both aesthetics and humor from a dialectical frame.

Returning to the Eastern philosophies, when the Zen Buddhist Master poses what would be to a demonstrative reasoner a contradiction-in-terms form of question – such as, 'what is the sound of one hand clapping? ' – he is making a dialectical point in his instruction (*Suzuki*, 1962). His aim here is to unite the student with the all-encompassing unity of nature. He is teaching that simply because one poses a question to be answered does not by that act legitimize the distinction implied by the question (leading to the break-up of nature into an artificial 'many' when nature is always a 'one'). Questions are asked by seekers, who often blind themselves to the very thing that they are seeking – i. e., a sense of the ultimate unity in being *(nirvana)*. Nature needs no questions, no scientific explanations. To experience the ultimate truth in nature, one must essentially slip into the round of totality in its spontaneous events and simply 'be' (the 'one' that nature is).

Conclusions and Plan of the Book

Our review has surely supported the opening claim that there can be no single meaning of dialectic for every theoretical account. If there is a core meaning in the dialectic, it would seem to be the idea of bipolarity, opposition, or contradiction. To be a true dialectic, one end of the bipolarity must diectly imply the other. The opposition cannot be artificial. For example, *Alfred Adler* once referred to dialectics in his approach as follows: 'It [dialectic] becomes apparent most often when we are dealing with persons who expect to be spoiled by others (thesis). When they do not receive such treatment, they fall into hate and resentment (antithesis), until they find their way through to contribution, to general humaneness (synthesis)' (*Ansbacher and Ansbacher*, 1964, p. 287). Although *Adler* has used the language of dialectic to frame his view, this is improper dialectic, because the thesis in this case (desire to be spoiled) is not truly an opposite implication or the contradiction of the antithesis cited (hatred for those who do not provide the spoiling). We cannot get a necessary implication of the latter from the former. The true opposite would be something quite different (fear of being spoiled, for example).

Once this meaning of the thesis implies or calls up its opposite, we have various ways in which the 'next' step (if any) is said to take place. Class-struggle ideas are likely to call for a victory of one side over the other, or, possibly some combining synthesis which calls up yet another thesis in the future. It is the movement from thesis-antithesis to synthesis concept which historians of developmental theoreticians in the social or psychological sciences like to emphasize. Often the concept of a 'new' or 'higher' level is suggested as, contradictions are worked out into new syntheses. But not all dialectical theories necessarily demand a resolution of contradictions. And surely not all of them require that this confrontation of opposite meanings in existence need someday come to an end. Whether or not syntheses take place, or final negations of negations occur, is up to the theorist making use of dialectical conceptions.

Our contention that the tie binding all dialectical formulations together is the inevitability of bipolarity in meaning (events, beliefs, classes, etc.) should not lead the reader to think that we mean there is one and *only* one antithesis to a given thesis. Even *Hegel* was known to postulate more than one antithesis to a thesis, allowing for *four* terms in the dialectical progression (*Stace,* 1955, p.97). But it is common for a person who hears about dialectic for the first time to give this conception an essentially demonstrative interpretation, thinking that what is meant by this opposition is some rigidly predictable A-versus-not-A tandem of a fixed (primary and true) duality. This is *not* what dialectical bipolarity means, of course. One person may have an implication to the opposite of a given thesis which is not premised by another person. This happens because what is affirmed in any given thesis is always some meaning expressed in a complex of potential meaning-extentions.

For example, to say 'Look for the lost watch down there, on the beach' expresses meanings of several varieties – both denotative and connotative. The statement itself takes on the intonation of a suggestion or even an order, so that one listener construing it in this fashion may sense immediately 'Why should I listen to you? ' and simply 'not look' as 'ordered'. A second person may challenge the 'primary and true' quality of the assumption that the watch has indeed been 'lost' and begin immediately such speculations as 'How do we know that the watch really is missing? ' And a third person can focus on the directions suggested and contemplate something like 'What makes you so certain it's down there on the beach, and not up here in the parking lot? ' Doubtless the reader can think of many other oppositional implications in this rather simple statement. And when we now add the factor of reasoning from an opposite to an opposite, we multiply the alternatives open to dialectical reasoning by a super-geometric ratio.

In order to introduce the reader to dialectical thinking in human description, as well as hopefully to recruit the reader into actual research on the dialectic (something we badly need), the plan of this book is to survey a number of different psychologists who are making use of the conception, allowing them to frame their particular usage in their own way. There are purely theoretical commentaries, but there are also chapters which get into the question of research on the dialectic as well as looking over extant research in light of this altered view of behavior. Empirical findings are cited in almost all of the chapters, so that there is a high standard of scholarship and scientific acumen reflected in these commentaries. Each chapter is a unit unto itself, and although it is really not possible to arrange the chapters into clear-cut sections, an ordering of sorts has been attempted.

We begin by looking at the dialectic as the often unnamed rationale for aesthetics (Chapter 2) and humor (Chapter 3). We then move to dialectical formulations of personality as suggested by psychoanalysis (Chapter 4) and its role in male-female relations (Chapter 5). The affinity which dialectical conceptions have for developmental theories then emerges in the next three chapters, which have to do respectively with moral development (Chapter 6), cognitive development (Chapter 7), and dialectical themes in Chinese culture (Chapter 8). We then move to a series of three chapters which look more directly at the process of scientific investigation and the findings which this process purports to discover. We take a look at the interpretation of the factual (Chapter 9), examine the possibility of a qualitative methodology (Chapter 10), and end the substantial chapters with a view of the subject in researches as a dialectician (Chapter 11). The closing chapter (12) of the volume then provides the reader with a summing up of what the entire volume has conveyed, and considers some of the reactions to and pitfalls in a dialectical approach to the science of behavior.

References

Adler, M. J.: Dialectic (Harcourt, Brace, New York 1927).

Adler, M. J. (ed.): The great ideas: a syntopicon; in *Hutchins* Great books of the western world, vol. 2, 3 (Encyclopedia Britannica, Chicago 1952).

Ansbacher, H. L. and Ansbacher, R. R. (ed.): Superiority and social interest (Northwestern University Press, Evanston 1964).

Aristotle: Physics, and Topics; in *Hutchins*, Great books of the western world, vol. 8. pp. 257–335, 143–223 (Encyclopedia Britannica, Chicago 1952).

Becker, H. and Barnes, H. E.: Social thought from lore to science (Harren Press, Washington 1952).

Burtt, E. A.: The metaphysical foundations of modern physical science; rev. ed. (Doubleday, Garden City 1955).

Freud, S.: The ego and the id, and other works; in *Strachey* The standard edition of the complete psychological works of Sigmund Freud, vol. XIX (Hogarth, London 1961).

Hauser, A.: The social history of art. Vol. I, Prehistoric, ancient-Oriental, Greece and Rome, middle ages; vol. II, Renaissance, mannerism, baroque; vol. III, Rococo, classicism, romanticism; vol. IV, Naturalism, impressionism, the film age (Vintage, New York 1951).

Hegel, G. W. F.: The philosophy of history, and The philosophy of right; in *Hutchins* Great books of the western world, vol. 46, pp. 153–369, 1–150 (Encyclopedia Britannica, Chicago 1952).

Hobbes, T.: Leviathan; in *Hutchins* Great books of the western world, vol. 23, pp. 49–283 (Encyclopedia Britannica, Chicago 1952).

Hook, S.: From Hegel to Marx (University of Michigan Press, Ann Arbor 1962).

Kant, I.: The critique of pure reason; in *Hutchins* Great books of the western world, vol. 42, pp. 1–250 (Encyclopedia Britannica, Chicago 1952).

Koffka, K.: Principles of gestalt psychology (Harcourt, Brace & World, New York 1935).

Kuhn, T. S.: The structure of scientific revolutions; 2nd ed. (University of Chicago Press, Chicago 1970).

Langer, S. K.: Philosophy in a new key (Penguin Books, New York 1948).

Locke, J.: An essay concerning human understanding; in *Hutchins* Great books of the western world, vol. 35, pp. 85–395 (Encyclopedia Britannica, Chicago 1952).

Magill, F. N. and McGreal, I. P.: Masterpieces of world philosophy, vol. I, II (Salem Press, New York 1961).
Marx, K.: Capital; in *Hutchins* Great books of the western world, vol. 50, pp. 1–393 (Encyclopedia Britannica, Chicago 1952).
McGuire, W. (ed.): The Freud / Jung letters: the correspondence between Sigmund Freud and C. G. Jung (Princeton University Press, Princeton 1974).
Moore, C. A.: The Chinese mind (East-West Center Press, Honolulu 1967a).
Moore, C. A.: The Indian mind (East-West Center Press, Honolulu 1967b).
Nākāmura, H.: Ways of thinking of eastern peoples: India-China-Tibet-Japan (East-West Center Press, Honolulu 1964).
Plato: Cratylus, Parmenides, Philebus, Sophist, and Statesman; in *Hutchins* Great books of the western world, vol. 7, pp. 85–639 (Encyclopedia Britannica, Chicago 1952).
Rychlak, J. F.: A philosophy of science for personality theory (Houghton Mifflin, Boston 1968).
Rychlak, J. F.: Introduction to personality and psychotherapy: a theory-construction approach (Houghton Mifflin, Boston 1973).
Stace, W. T.: The philosophy of Hegel (Dover, New York 1955).
Suzuki, D. T.: The essentials of Zen Buddhism; in *Phillips* (Dutton, New York 1962).

Contr. hum. Dev., vol. 2, pp. 18–25 (Karger, Basel 1976)

Chapter 2
The Dialectic as an Approach to Psychological Aesthetics

Robert J. Sardello

There are several ways to approach art from the psychological perspective. It is possible to engage in a psychology of the creative act, as for example the work of *Weber* (1969). It is possible to begin with a consideration of the art object as does *Vygotsky* (1971). It is possible to focus on the image of man present in art (*Rychlak*, 1968). Finally, it is possible to concentrate on the relation between the observer of art and the art object, as in the work of *Berlyne* (1971). There are, of course, intrinsic relations among these alternatives, but the focus of this chapter will be primarily on the aesthetic experience *per se.*

Even though the dialectical view of meaning can aid tremendously in the understanding of the peculiarly human phenomenon we term aesthetic experience, psychology has persisted in viewing such 'behavior' in exclusively demonstrative terms (see Chapter 1). As we begin to make explicit the role of dialectic in psychology, we therefore find that we must begin with the existing mode of thought, understand the merits and limits of this mode, and then begin to pose an alternative way of conceptualizing our area of interest. I contend that a dialectical approach to aesthetics will not only provide an immediate rationale for a more humanistic psychology, but it will enable the investigator in this area to account for the aesthetic experience in a more accurate, hence instructive manner.

Psychological aesthetics is one of the oldest areas of experimental psychology. It is also one of the most confused. In his *Aesthetics and Psychobiology*, *Berlyne* (1971) has attempted to place psychological aesthetics on firm behavioristic ground. An extremely important presupposition pervades the thinking of that book. A work of art or an art object is said to be a system of signs. *Berlyne* (1971, p. 53) defines a sign as an object or event from which stimuli originate and which stands for some other object. Following the philosopher *Morris*, *Berlyne* (1971, p. 56) defines a symbol as a stimulus that is a sign for the organism producing it. This way of talking about the symbolic character of art alludes to the necessity of a concern for awareness or experience, or contemplation, but in such a way that interiority does not really have to be faced and dealt with. By reducing symbol to sign, the way is clear to speak only of external relations between sign and organism in efficient-causal fashion. This is precisely what *Berlyne* proceeds to do.

According to *Berlyne* (1971, pp. 137–174), when a person is confronted with an art object, he is confronted with a system of signs. These stimuli vary along certain measurable dimensions, namely psychophysical, ecological, and most importantly, collative dimensions. Collative stimuli are qualitatively complex stimuli involving past meaning and perception of form. *Berlyne*'s concept of arousal in relation to aesthetic experience is based on a physicalist view of perception. This view of perception assumes that when we see things aesthetically our attention is directed to the way in which the thing is presented – as novel, as complex and so on – rather than to the integrity of the 'thing' as such. The measurement of arousal in relation to perceptual objects in the laboratory which are supposed to vary along the dimensions of collative variables such as novelty and complexity amounts to an unwarranted abstraction from such artificial procedures. In aesthetic experience I may indeed be confronted with a complex thing or a novel thing. For example, if we look at Van Gogh's painting of peasant's shoes we see that we cannot tell where the shoes stand. There is nothing surrounding this pair of peasant shoes in or to which they might belong. There is only an undefined space. This is indeed a novel way to see shoes.

But, what happens when I try to abstract the novelty from the shoes. I take what is proper to this aesthetic experience – a novel view of shoes – and make novelty into a sign which has an effect on an organism. This sign (abstract novelty) is then made the cause of an emotion with a given state of activation or arousal. Thus, account is taken of two of the most important qualities in an aesthetic experience – i. e., perception and emotion – but at the cost of making these qualities extrinsic to each other and then postulating a causal relation between them. Yet, when I look at Van Gogh's painting of the peasant's shoes I am struck by the novel shoes, not *solely* by the novelty. To understand the painting I must contemplate the shoes in and of themselves. The 'novel shoes' are of a symbolic character, not simply a sign varying along the dimension of novelty which produces a level of arousal. *Heidegger* (1964, p. 663) explicates the density of meaning of those shoes as follows:

> From the dark opening of the worn insides of the shoes the toilsome thread of the worker stands forth. In the stiffly solid heaviness of the shoes there is the accumulated tenacity of her slow trudge through the far-spreading and ever uniform furrows of the field. On the leather lies the dampness and saturation of the soil. Under the soles there slides the loneliness of the field-path as the evening declines. In the shoes there vibrates the silent call of the earth, its quiet gift of the ripening corn and its enigmatic self-refusal in the fallow desolation of the wintery field.

The painting of the peasant's shoes must be understood as a symbolic expression *in complexio*. A symbol is a sign, but it is much more. A sign always reveals a one-to-one correspondence. A sign refers to something beyond itself which is definite and specific. A red light on the highway is a sign which means stop. A symbol also refers to something beyond itself; however, it refers not to a single referent but rather to an inexhaustible realm of meaning (*Royce*, 1965). The shoes in Van Gogh's painting do not have a single referent, but have the world of meaning suggested by *Heidegger*. Furthermore, we can speak of a symbol whenever something objective and subjective, something 'external' and 'inward' have been fused into a concrete sensuous representation (*Caligor and May*, 1968). The peasant's shoes are shoes, but they are simultaneously toil and trudge and loneliness. A psychological aesthetics must be able to deal with the symbolic realm on its own terms. A reduction of the symbolic realm to the realm of signs is not precisely wrong, but it is severely limiting.

'Sign' as a Demonstrative Construct

In a psychobiological account of the aesthetic experience, the reason a symbolic realm is reduced to the realm of signs is because a sign is a surface phenomenon while a symbol is a depth phenomenon. I 'see' surfaces spread out before me. When knowledge is likened to sight, knowing becomes almost exclusively a matter of explanation (ex-planare – to lay out flat, to open up), a laying out on a surface to present maximum exteriority. The relation between sign, stimulus, arousal, and hedonic value is plain and clear. This explanation of aesthetic experience presents a distinctness, an edge, a precision and clarity, qualities like those paramount in vision. The sign has no depth. It points to a single referent in a flat, linear manner.

However, the symbolic realm is not capable of being understood through the visual analogue because the symbolic realm is one of depth, multiplicity, and interiority. The symbolic realm has a certain denseness, a certain opacity. To illustrate, let us use an example from *Ricoeur*'s (1967) work *The Symbolism of Evil*. He tells us that the word 'impure' is a symbol which refers beyond itself and means 'stained' (*Ricoeur*, 1967, pp. 14–18). The first sign which is literal, itself points to a second meaning – a situation of man in relation to the sacred. Further, this situation of man as defiling the sacred is inexhaustible; that is, there are many meanings of man as defiling which cannot be fully or immediately transparent.

The demonstrative metaconstruct of stimulus-response which relies so heavily on the visual analogue cannot approach an understanding of the aesthetic experience of human beings. Understanding is not like seeing. Understanding grows with time. I understand one point, then another, and a third, often in contradiction to the second, and so forth. Understanding changes as I move from the first point to the second, and so on. Knowledge of aesthetic experience is not typically perfected by the qualities adequate to vision, such as distinctness, precision, and clarity.

The Dialectical Nature of Aesthetic Experience

Sound provides an even more appropriate analogue to construct development in psychological aesthetics than does vision. *Ong* (1967 pp. 117–118), in *The Presence of the Word*, says that sound better represents the world of dynamism, action, and being-in-time:

> Sound . . . reveals the interior without the necessity of physical invasion. Thus we tap a wall to discover whether it is perhaps lead inside. To discover such things by sight, we should have to open what we examine, making the inside the outside, destroying its interiority as such. Sound reveals interiors because its nature is determined by interior relationships.

Vision or sight permits us to assimilate inanimate 'things' to our knowledge very directly, whereas to know a 'person' we must perforce enter into the sensory realm of hearing. Speaking with another to communicate involves a dialogue, a give-and-take as each side comes to understand the meaningful implications of the other. Indeed, one side determines the meaning direction of the other and vice versa in a truly open dialogue (i. e., in which the participants are sincere, responsive one to the other, etc.). This is clearly a dialectical process. I would like to suggest that just as a person to whom we relate dialectically in this fashion presents us with a certain opacity calling for the give-and-take of dialogue, so too does the symbolic representations of an art object present the observer with a certain opacity needing clarification in the *subjective* relationship between the art work and the observer. In this sense, an art object is more than a 'thing'; it is an 'expressing thing' calling for dialectical examination and personal, subjective clarification by an observer. Of course, it is true in principle that objective communication is possible, so that one person – the art critic – might speak for all of us as he 'communicates with' the work of art. But the essence of art, its richness, is the subjective variations possible – variations which are only clarified when we grasp the fact that this is a dialectical process. Artists and art critics seem more aware of this than psychologists, since they often say that the art work 'speaks to them'. We might add that they usually 'answer', infusing the work with a richness that was sometimes not recognized by the artist. *Hegel*'s conception of *alienation* takes root from this idea that a work of art can stand free of its creator, and enter into new dialogues, expressing meanings never intended by its creator – who is now alienated from his intent (assuming he had one; i. e., not all artists create to convey a fixed message; *Paolucci and Paolucci,* 1962).

Thus, the aesthetic experience is not a fixed state, a response to some immediately discernible entity. The 'perception-to-emotion' sequence in aesthetic experience is not efficiently 'cause-effect', but rather one of 'thesis-antithesis-synthesis', with an ever-expanding course of meaning induction and enrichment as a possibility (i. e., it need *not* occur). As *Muller-Vollmer* (1963) notes, feelings demand a 'reflective presence' to the world insofar as we refer to the feelings of human beings. We cannot feel without wanting to express, to reflect once again on that which provoked this feeling in our awareness. This brings us into a dialectical confrontation with art objects, which is the fundamental aspect – the very core! – of the aesthetic experience. If we permit it to develop, we are brought ever more into a state of aesthetic *contemplation*.

What are some of the dimensions of aesthetic contemplation? Aesthetic contemplation first of all involves the dialectic of active participation and passive observation. I look at Van Gogh's painting of the peasant's shoes and I *must* become involved with the painting to such a degree that I have feelings about those shoes, the toil and drudgery and loneliness of those shoes. At the same time, this belief does not go so far as to coincide with the real. I do not attempt to pick the shoes up and try them on. At this point I am passively observing the shoes, cognizant of their symbolic meanings.

In the realm of contemplation these attitudes of active participation and passive observation can exist together without being contradictory. *Lynch* (1965) points out that such fundamental bipolar oppositions existed in harmony for ages until the gnostics saw no possibility of reconciliation between oppositional ideas. The resultant conflict in their ideology represents the shift in history from contemplation to logical knowing, with the attendant analogue of vision to knowing (see above). From the Greeks to the gnostics, reality was seen as containing the odd and even, the masculine and feminine, the light and dark, the one and many. The gnostics put these principles into battle – light versus dark, a world of eternal life without decay or death versus death without eternal life, and so on.

A second dimension of aesthetic contemplation is the dialectic of subjective-objective. I bring my own individual, lived history to the art work and relate that history to the work. As *Weber* (1969) says, I project myself sympathetically into the work. At the same time it is necessary to resist this subjective temptation to experience the work the way in which 'I' want to experience it, and, rather, to contemplate 'what is there', i. e., to assume a more objective attitude. The importance and difficulty of this attitude are emphasized and assisted by the art critic or the literary critic. Such critics help us to recognize subjective responses and aid us in returning to a consideration of the work itself.

For example, one can read *Faulkner*'s (1959) novel *Light in August* and be attracted by the love story of Lena Grove and Byron Bunch, the story of a man finding his beautiful lady. Or, one can be attracted to the novel because it is the story of the friendship between Byron Bunch and Gail Hightower, the relation between a young man and an old man that seems to be fruitful for both. Finally, one may be attracted to the Joe Christmas story in the novel. This is the story of a man estranged from nature, from his past, and from others. The totality of the work, as pointed out by the literary critic *Brooks* (1971, p. 179) is the community, the great counterforce to which the characters are attracted or against which they are reacting:

> But for many a reader, the community is indeed invisible and quite imperceptible; it exerts no pressure on him at all – and lacking any awareness of this force, he may miss the meaning of the work. Such readers find *Light in August* quite baffling simply because they are unaware of the force of community that pervades it and thus miss the clue to its central structure.

Again, the subjective-objective dialectic is not contradictory in the realm of contemplation. Both attitudes occur simultaneously and are in harmony in aesthetic experience.

A further dialectic of aesthetic contemplation is the relation of art to artist. When I confront a work of art I contemplate the meaning of the work itself, what vision of life is being articulated or what expression of reality is represented. At the same time, I question and wonder what the artist intended and how he came to produce such a work. This reflects a spontaneous belief that it is the artist's lived experience which provides the substance of his work. *Muller-Vollmer* (1963) points out that the philosopher *Wilhelm Dilthey* had this view of the relation of art to experience. For *Dilthey* all literature is somehow built from concrete life-experience. Even poets who have presented purely imaginary worlds have had to depend on actual representations and life-experiences for their sensory imagery. This must mean that an understanding of the artist's life can enhance the meaning of his work for the observer. At the same time, it is impossible to reduce the art work to the intention of the artist. As noted above in the reference to alienation, the art work has a life of its own.

In the past, some critics have tended to reduce the work of art to the life of the artist, and in particular to the psychological difficulties of the artist. *Jung* (1933) found this approach to be severely limiting to the understanding of art because all such an approach elucidates is that artists are as human as the rest of us. As a reaction against leaving the art work to speak of the art work, the cry of the Southern literary critics such as *Allen Tate* and *John Crowe Ransom* was to return to the work itself. These critics argue that the meaning of the work of art is present in the totality of the work, but requires an awakening to the sense of totality. Both *Jung* and the Southern literary critics present, then, formalizations of the sides of the fundamental paradox of the relation between the art work and the artist. The work of art carries the life of the artist and simultaneously moves beyond that individual life.

Wimsatt (1958) has beautifully documented one last dimension of aesthetic contemplation that I would like to consider here. *Wimsatt* calls this dimension the 'concrete universal', a term taken from *Hegel* which refers to the fact that when I encounter a work of art I confront a very individual thing and at the same time a very universal thing. This is the paradox of how universality can be made communicable through a sensuous medium other than the abstract sign system of purely rational, logical discourse. I look at a painting of a rose. It is a very individualistic rose, a beautiful rose with concave petals reaching toward the sun, emanating a glow. At the same time that rose expresses a world of meaning . . . the feminine, the unfolding of life, power, seductive beauty, and so on. Neither of these polarities can be forgotten. To experience only the individual rose is to flatten and truncate the experience.

Again, this dialectic of individual aesthetic contemplation has been formalized on both sides by critics and philosophers. *Wimsatt* (1958, p. 395) points out that *Samuel Johnson* emphasizes the universal, recognizing that figures in literature are not modified by the customs of particular places, or by peculiarities of situation or by temporary opinions. They are the progeny of common humanity. On the other hand, *Henri Bergson* emphasizes the particular, arguing that art always aims at what is individual; what the artist expresses is something he has seen at a certain hour on a certain day that will never be again. In individual aesthetic contemplation, both sides of this dialectic exist in harmonious integration.

The Human Reality

These dimensions of the dialectic of aesthetic contemplation help us to realize that an aesthetic presence to the world does involve contradictories and opposites, but in the aesthetic experience these contradictories are not experienced as conflictual. The symbolic realm is precisely where there can exist a harmony of contradiction (many among one). The existence of one polarity does not demand the denying or the killing-off of another. This paradoxical character of human reality becomes increasingly apparent as we attempt to understand the more uniquely human modes of experience. Contrary to *Berlyne* (1971), I do not think that animals – even monkeys – are capable of aesthetic experience. *Köhler*'s (1925) work with chimpanzees has shown us that animals do think, but only man thinks symbolically. Only man, then, is capable of the awe, wonder, contemplation, admiration and appreciation we recognize as the aesthetic experience.

References

Berlyne, D. E.: Aesthetics and psychobiology (Appleton Century Crofts, New York 1971).

Brooks, C.: The community and the pariah; in *Vickery and Vickery* Light in August and the critical spectrum, p. 175–196 Belmont (Wadsworth, 1971).

Caligor, L. and May, R.: Dreams and symbols (Basic Books, New York 1968).

Faulkner, W.: Light in August (Modern Library, New York 1959).

Heidegger, M.: The origin of the work of art; in *Hofstader and Kuhns* Philosophies of art and beauty, pp. 649–701 (Modern Library and Random House, New York, 1964).

Jung, C. G.: Psychology and literature; in Modern man in search of a soul, pp. 152–173; transl. by Dell and Baynes (Harcourt, Brace & World, New York 1933).

Köhler, W.: The mentality of apes; transl. by Winters (Routledge & Kegan, London 1925).

Lynch, W.: Images of hope (New American Library, New York 1965).

Muller-Vollmer, K.: Towards a phenomenological theory of literature (Mouton, The Hague 1963).

Ong, W.: The presence of the word (Simon & Schuster, New York 1967).

Paolucci, A. and Paolucci, H.: Hegel: on tragedy (Doubleday, Garden City 1962).

Ricoeur, P.: The symbolism of evil; transl. by Buchanan (Harper & Row, New York 1967).

Royce, J. R.: Psychology at the crossroads; in *Royce* Psychology and the symbol, pp. 3–25 (Random House, New York 1965).

Rychlak, J. F.: A philosophy of science for personality theory (Houghton Mifflin, Boston 1968).

Vygotsky, L. S.: The psychology of art (MIT Press, Cambridge 1971).

Weber, J. P.: The psychology of art (Delta Books, New York 1969).

Wimsatt, W. K.: The structure of the 'concrete universal' in literature; in *Schorer, Miles and McKenzie* Criticism, p. 393–407 (Harcourt, Brace & World, New York 1958).

Contr. hum. Dev., vol. 2, pp. 26–33 (Karger, Basel 1976)

Chapter 3
Dialectics and the Psychology of Laughter

Robert J. Sardello

As an approach to psychology, dialectics not only examines behavior through bipolarities in meaning, its questioning procedures follow a dialogical mode of thought (see Chapter 1). This mode of thought always attempts to locate its questions 'on the other side' of taken-for-granted apprehensions. For this reason, dialecticians seem to like controversy and appear to enjoy being critical or argumentative. Actually, it is not obstinance that motivates this mode of thinking, but simply the attempt to keep thought alive. Where there is unity, the dialectical thinker will find diversity. Where there is diversity, the dialectical thinker will find unity.

This paper will examine humor and laughing, an area of psychology which is itself filled with diversity of opinion, and will seek to find an expression of unity within such multiplicity of viewpoints. Further, this unity will not be sought in some overarching theoretical construct which pretends to be able to unite what is divided, but will simply state that there is 'another side' to this multiplicity of opinion. The finding of this 'other side' is already a dialectical operation. The dialectic will be doubled, however, as we discover that the very nature of humor and laughing consists of dialectical action.

Theories of Humor as a Laughing Matter

We could easily devote this chapter to a review of the numerous theories of humor and laughing. *Bergler* (1956) summarizes no less than 80 such theories. Whose theory are we to believe? It is a testimony to the richness of this phenomenon that so many diverse and competing theories have been proposed. We shall have to immerse ourselves in some of this diversity in order to experience the unity which is *also* there. Rather than survey the 80 theories summarized by *Bergler*, a more recent and useful classification for our purposes has been proposed by *Keith-Spiegel* (1972). She has organized the existing theories into eight fundamental types.

1. Evolutionary and group theories. McDougall (1903) views laughter as having evolved as a balance to sympathy. Primitive man lived a group life in which he was constantly immersed in the feelings of the group. Laughter allows a release and thus the ability to separate from others. *McComas* (1923) and *Hayworth* (1928) theorized that laughter is a remnant of an adaptive signal behavior that used to indicate to a group that danger had passed. Laughter originated as a social warning device. *Ludovici* (1932) argued that laughter was a relic of struggling, biting, and physical attack. Attack and ridicule originates laughter in man.

These theories concern themselves with origins. They suggest that an origin remains always with what it originates and what is originated sustains this kernal source. Evolutionary and group theories, therefore, express the fact that a primitive element resides at the heart of our being. Humor and laughter are expressions of our bodily life, our life prior to reflection, our life of feeling. Even so, laughing as a release from others is a primitive expression of opposition, of being different and 'other than the group'.

2. Superiority theories. Cooper (1922) pointed out that *Aristotle* understood humor and laughter as arising from a sense of triumph over others. Whenever we perceive weaknesses in others or the sufferings of others we are led to laughter. Many other theorists have framed a similar understanding (*Hobbes*, 1952; *Sidis*, 1913; *Wallis*, 1922). The 'laugher' is expressing superiority over the 'one laughed at'. This attitude of superiority is also an expression of difference. The superior person is 'above' others, resulting in a separation not unlike that of the evolutionary and group theories as regards interpersonal relations.

3 and 4. Incongruity and surprise theories. Schopenhauer (1819), *Spencer* (1860), *Bergson* (1908), and *Koestler* (1964) have all expressed the idea that laughter arises from ideas or events that are illogical, divergent, or contradictory to one another. *Stanley* (1898), *Hobbes* (1952), *Sully* (1902), *Fiebleman* (1939), and *Berlyne* (1972) all consider surprise as necessary for humor and laughter to develop. Surprise means that there is a discontinuity with the normal.

All of the theories mentioned so far can be understood as saying that humor and laughing concern the perception of the fact that things are not what they seem. The evolutionary and group theories express that all is not encompassed by primitive group life. The superiority theories state that everyone is not the same. Incongruity and surprise theories directly express the fact that things simultaneously are and are not as they seem.

5 and 6. Release, relief, and psychoanalytic theories. Spencer (1860) argued that laughter is the release of physical energy. *Grieg* (1923) argued that laughter is the release of psychological energy, and *Menon* (1931) argued for laughter as the release of emotional energy. Psychoanalytic theories also employ the metaphor of energy. For *Freud* (1905), laughter is a release of psychic energy which is not allowed to discharge in more direct ways because of the watchfulness of the superego. Laughter is a disguised outlet of the original impulse.

Energy metaphors place emphasis on the admitted physical, bodily side to humor and laughter. If humor and laughter express the cognitive fact that things are not as they seem, then metaphors of energy express the parallel fact that this perception is not simply conceptual, but involves the immediacy of our felt bodily participation in the world and with others.

7 and 8. Ambivalence and configurational theories. Ambivalence theories are very similar to incongruity theories; however, they locate incongruity at the level of emotion rather than ideas. For *Joubert* (*Eastman*, 1921), laughing is the incongruity between joy and sorrow; for *Grieg* (1923), love and hate; for *Winterstein* (1934), mania and depression; for *Dessoir* (1923), superiority and imitation; for *Gregory* (1924), sympathy and animosity; and for *Knox* (1951), playfulness and seriousness. Configurational theories are also like incongruity theories in stressing a cognitive element. However, configurational theorists stress the sense of things falling into place rather than the reverse sense of a disjointedness in things (*Wallis*, 1922; *Maier*, 1932). *McGhee* (1972) developed a configurational theory that emphasized the total relation of the laughter with the object, and thus included both emotion and cognition.

It is clear that configurational and ambivalence theories of humor and laughter simply find another way of expressing the dialectical relationship within events that we have seen emerging in all of the other theories. The fundamental theme continues to be that things are both what they seem to be and yet are unlike what they seem to be. One cannot find this duality in an objective assessment of some 'fact pattern', but rather we know it by way of the recurring duality of our bodily involvement in a succession of lived situations which are never one, but are many in the implications they engender. The tie binding all theories of humor is therefore the dialectical metaconstruct.

The Dialectics of Laughing and Humor

Human beings are constantly emersed in situations which have a dual character. There is no love without hate, no power without innocence (*May*, 1971), no here without there, no up without down, no day without night, or no joy without sorrow. And yet, we are not always laughing. Laughter can occur only when we pay attention. We have to expect the unexpected for humor and laughter to come to expression. Children are always laughing because they constantly live in an attitude of wonder. When we pay attention in an attitude of wonder, then there is the perception and discovery that things are not what they seem and are what they seem not to be. *Verhoven* (1972, p. 27) speaks of wonder as the 'experience of self between establishing that a reality is thus and that it is different, the melting point between liquidity or evaporation and opacity or petrification. Confronting reality at this point is the state of suspension between the grasped and the ungrasped. It is one and the other or neither one nor the other, never one without the other'.

Laughing originates in an intolerable situation that one, through the attitude of wonder, allows to be intolerable and to which one pays attention. Even more important, laughing occurs when one establishes a certainty about what is and what is not in attention, and then suddenly throws this established illusion into question. For example, one of my students wrote the following description of a situation in which she found herself laughing:

> A Sunday evening. I had watched a TV program with the family. Toward the end I told our son to get ready for bed during a commercial because it would be ten o'clock when the program was over, and that is his bedtime. As soon as the program was over I told him to get to bed (several times) and finally maneuvered him into his bedroom. I prepared the kitchen for breakfast the next morning, told my daughter good-night, then went to our older son and told him good-night. He said, 'At nine o'clock? ' At first I didn't believe him, but it was indeed nine instead of ten. Not only had I gotten myself ready for bed one hour early – I'm usually late – but I had also gotten our 14 year old to bed early – and he hurries to bed like a turtle on a hot summer day! I thought the situation was funny.
>
> I was thinking, what a joke on me – how dumb to think it was an hour later than it was. I felt silly and laughed at myself. It was a big hearty laugh coming from somewhere deep inside. It kept coming – sort of an effervescence. I felt the physical, chuckling feeling inside me. It felt similar to someone uncorking a bottle of champagne and the bubbles escaping. It was a feeling of release. A happy feeling. The laughter sort of took possession of my body and left me feeling 'limp' while I was laughing – somewhat helpless.

We can summarize the meaning of this situation of laughing as follows: A humorous situation can occur when the rapidness and determinedness of our everyday thinking are stopped cold in their tracks. In fulfilling her responsibilities as a good mother, the person in this protocol is constantly working out situations in advance. In our lived experience, this type of thinking is crucial if we are to pass through each day smoothly and on to the next. But when this constant flow is abruptly halted and thrown back upon us, it comes to be seen in a new light. When the continuity of everyday life is shattered, a queer feeling of disorientation creeps over us. When we finally regain our bearing and discover that by constructing situations as we think they should be in advance, we have led ourselves into a foolish situation, the feeling of what we later name irony, and futility in our position gives us a new perspective on things. We find ourselves stepping outside the ordinary pre-reflective view of lived events to a cognitive realization of this irony and futility, as well as the innocent playfulness and foolishness which are a part of this situation. Without this move to a new view, the situation will remain merely absurd, irrational, and even unfair.

But once the step to the new view has been taken, we laugh at ourselves and the situation we led ourselves into. Our stupidity or the ridiculous nature of our actions no longer seems important as the laughing takes full possession of our being. Thus, humor and laughing are fundamentally dialectical experiences. Laughing is a saying 'No' to an assumed 'Yes'. A previously assumed familiarity is suddenly reversed. On the other hand, dialectics is that possibility of saying 'Yes' to an assumed 'No'. The following protocol from another student illustrates the other side of this yes-no dialectic:

> One time when I laughed so very hard was when I did something that was way below my intelligence and age level. I walked into my bedroom and for no reason that I can possibly think of, I ran and jumped on the bed on my head and rolled off the other side of the bed after almost breaking my neck.
>
> My roommate saw me do this and she started laughing at me. I, too, laughed so hard that I cried. While I was laughing, I was wondering what made me do such a childish thing. At that moment I felt so carefree and lighthearted and happy. I was also somewhat embarrassed that someone saw me do such a thing as that. But the feeling of real hearty laughter made me forget everything else for just a few minutes. My whole being was engrossed in the feeling. When I finally quit laughing so hard, I felt totally relaxed but tired. My mind was relaxed also, which is a rare happening.

This humorous situation is characterized by a spontaneity – an action without any felt reason or cause. The events which unfold into instances of humor need no rational provocation for their occurrence. Though these actions may be in direct conflict with what is supposed to be going on, they need no justification and can happen in situations where they are uncalled for and even forbidden. The person in this situation plunged head-long into the absurd and became saturated with it. She found herself submerged in the world of the ridiculous and temporarily threw off all objective considerations. However, she became conscious that what she was doing was absurd. Once this happened, the world around her tried to pull her out of the absurdity of the situation as she felt childish and embarrassed about what she had done. But she was already enveloped by her inner feelings of lightness and happiness.

In the dialectic of laughing and humor, a 'conversation' is initiated with the opposite side of ourselves. These conversations never reach a definite conclusion. Certainty and familiarity are thrown into uncertainty and surprise. The second situation described above in which there was a saying 'No' to the familiar is perhaps closer to tragedy, but this simply indicates the close relationship between the comic and the tragic. The clown image provides us with an example of this closeness between comedy and tragedy. *Griffith* (1966, pp. 96–97) describes a scene from a movie of that greatest clown of all, Charlie Chaplin:

> In the film, 'The Gold Rush,' possibly his greatest, Charlie Chaplin is reduced to eating one of his famous shoes. What respect he pays it. He eats with overstyled gestures, winding the shoelace-spaghetti around his fork, mincing the last morsel from each nail-bone. This scene would not have been as funny had he eaten his hat, we can be sure of that, for the hidden motif throughout the film, the chord for all his tunes, is the foot. The Alaskan climate requires that he replace the shoe he's eaten. He wraps his foot with layer upon layer of burlap, making it more cumbersome than before. This is the film in which he gave his inspired bread dance, the dance which may contain the purest image of the clown. He sinks forks into two dinner rolls shaped like submarines. These fork-legs and bun-feet frolic in a way in which he could not ... Toward the end of the film, with the suddenness and the contradiction which marks the humorous, he kicks his gross sack-foot against his backside from the knee. It is as though the foot acted flippantly on its own as an abrupt denial of heaviness and inarticulation, it brings the audience into the fun as though the foot had turned to us and winked.

Thus, we see another dimension to the dialectic of laughter. Laughter and humor are both comic and tragic. This way of speaking of laughing is called irony. In irony there is no longer the duality of the serious and the not serious. Laughter is tragicomic, which is ironic. For this reason, the ability to laugh at oneself is therapeutic and laughing is essentially following the dictum 'know thyself'. We are what we are not. Laughter may indeed be the most profound dialectic of all.

Laughing and the Body

In the descriptions of laughing provided above we see that the dialectic of laughing is formed in bodily expression. Laughing is a form of expression, but it is unlike other forms of expression such as language or gesture. In laughing we lose control; an objective manipulation of the lived situation is temporarily suspended. Laughing surges from the life of feeling. It is characterized by an eruptivity and a compulsiveness. Laughing is a physical reaction unlike other physical reactions such as blushing or turning pale. The latter are passive reactions to situations, whereas laughing is a reaction to a situation which presents itself to a person as a problem, but as a problem which is unsolvable.

Plessner (1970), in a work entitled *Laughing and Crying*, offers an understanding of laughing based on the relation of the person to his body. *Plessner* points out that we usually respond to situations as persons. Without getting into the problem of what we mean by a person, what is meant here is that ordinarily we take our body for granted. We respond to situations as persons and make use of our body for that purpose. But, according to *Plessner* (1970, pp. 65–69), we do not always live our body as the incarnation of our existence in situations. Man is unique in being the only animal to live a dual relation to his body; he both *is* a body and *has* a body. This simultaneous being and having a body *Plessner* terms 'eccentricity'. The eccentric position of man means that he is not totally merged in being a body nor having a body. Man is neither just a living body, nor does he just have a body. Furthermore, we are aware of the ambiguous relation of being and having a body.

Man is aware of his physical situation. We live the constant 'problem' of being and having a body. Typically, the situation smoothly offers the possible response so that the 'problem' goes unnoticed. For example, I can utilize my body to move about, carry loads, sit, grasp, lie, and so on. In other situations I can deliberately control my body to execute a response. Sometimes, however, if the situation is threatening to the self, the dialectical relation of being and having a body, which constitutes the integrity of the person, breaks down and a person either retreats from his body, a psychotic-like response, or merges totally into being a body, i. e., behaves erratically and to no purpose.

If the situation is not seen as threatening, the integrity of the person is maintained by temporarily giving up 'having' a body and allowing the body to solve the 'problem' for him. Laughing is the solution the body gives. *Plessner* (1970, pp. 66–68) writes:

> By slipping as if by accident into the physical process and giving way to it, a process opaque in itself which runs its course compulsively, by the disorganization of his inner balance, man at once forfeits the relation to his body *and* re-establishes it. The effective impossibility of finding a suitable expression and an appropriate answer is at the same time the only suitable expression, the only appropriate answer . . . the body takes over the gesture, or expressive movement, but as body. In losing control over his body . . . he still knows how to find an answer.

Viewed from the perspective of the body, laughing expresses the dialectical relation of being and having a body maintaining the expression of being a person.

While we may seem to have provided two explanations of laughing and humor, one culminating with the notion of irony and the other culminating in our bodily life as persons, these accounts merge into each other. Both explanations rely on a fundamental dialectic, but express that there are levels in this dialectic of laughing. Considered at the level of a situation, laughing is the expression of living with an attitude of wonder in which the unfamiliar is found in the familiar and vice versa. Considered at the level of our response to situations, laughing is the expression of being directed to situations as persons. If the first account finally takes us to philosophy, then the second account finally takes us to psychology.

References

Bergler, E.: Laughter and the sense of humor (Intercontinental Medical Book, New York, 1956).

Bergson, H.: Laughter: an essay on the meaning of comic (Macmillan, New York 1908).

Berlyne, D.: Humor and its kin; in *Goldstein and McGhee* The psychology of humor, pp. 43–99 (Academic Press, New York 1972).
Cooper, L.: An Aristotelian theory of comedy (Harcourt, New York 1922).
Dessoir, M.: Ästhetik und allgemeine Kunstwissenschaft (Enke, Stuttgart 1923).
Eastman, M.: The sense of humor (Scribners, New York 1921).
Fiebleman, J. K.: In praise of comedy (Macmillan, New York 1939).
Freud, S.: Der Witz und seine Beziehung zum Unbewussten (Leipzig / Vienna, 1905).
Gregory, J. C.: The nature of laughter (Kegan, London 1924).
Grieg, J. Y. T.: The psychology of laughter and comedy (Dodd, Mead, New York 1923).
Griffith, R.: Anthropodology: man a-foot; in *von Bayer and Griffith* Conditio humana, pp. 84–102 (Springer, New York 1966).
Hayworth, D.: The social origins and functions of laughter. Psychol. Rev. *35* 367–384 (1928).
Hobbes, T.: Leviathan; in *Hutchins* Great books of the western world; vol. 23, pp. 49–283 (Encyclopedia Britannica, Chicago 1952).
Keith-Spiegel, P.: Early conceptions of humor: varieties and issues; in *Goldstein and McGhee* The psychology of humor, pp. 4–34 (Academic Press, New York 1972).
Knox, I.: Towards a philosophy of humor. J. Phil. *48:* 541–548 (1951).
Koestler, A.: The act of creation (Hutchinson, London 1964).
Ludovici, A. M.: The secret of laughter (Constable, London 1932).
Maier, N. R. F.: A gestalt theory of humor. B. J. Psychol. *23:* 69–74 (1932).
May, R.: Power and innocence (Norton, New York 1971).
McComas, H. C.: The origin of laughter. Psychol. Rev. *30:* 45–55 (1923).
McDougall, W.: The theory of laughter. Nature, Lond. *67:* 318–319 (1903).
McGhee, P.: On the cognitive origins of incongruity humor: fantasy assimilation versus reality assimilation; in *Goldstein and McGhee* The psychology of humor, pp. 61–79 (Academic Press, New York 1972).
Menon, V. K.: A theory of laughter (Allen & Unwin, London 1931).
Plessner, H.: Laughing and crying: a study of the limits of behavior (Northwestern University Press, Evanston 1970).
Schopenhauer, A.: Die Welt als Wille und Vorstellung (Brockhaus, Leipzig 1819).
Sidis, B.: The psychology of laughter (Appleton, New York 1913).
Spencer, H.: The physiology of laughter. Macmillan's Mag. *1:* 395–402 (1860).
Stanley, H. M.: Remarks on tickling and laughing. Am. J. Psychol. *9:* 235–240 (1898).
Sully, J.: Essay on laughter (Longmans Green, New York 1902).
Verhoven, N.: The philosophy of wonder (Macmillan, New York 1972).
Wallis, W. O.: 'Why do we laugh? ' Scient. Mon., N. Y. *15:* 343–347 (1922).
Winterstein, A.: Contributions to the problem of humor. Psychoanal. Q. *3:* 303–316 (1934).

Contr. hum. Dev., vol. 2, pp. 34–43 (Karger, Basel 1976)

Chapter 4
Sigmund Freud: The Reluctant Dialectician

Joseph F. Rychlak

Sometime late in 1892, *Freud* (1966 a) drafted a paper entitled 'A case of successful treatment by hypnotism', publishing it even before he and *Breuer* published their 'Preliminary Communication' (*Breuer and Freud,* 1955), which is the paper usually cited as *Freud*'s very first theoretical effort. In the latter paper we find *Breuer* and *Freud* speaking of hysteria as due to *strangulated affects*; i. e., emotional reactions, which have never been made, that are now cut-off from the rest of mind and lending havoc to the personality. Such dammed-up emotions must be released through *abreactions* (i. e., hypnotic relivings of the long-forgotten situation in which the affect was strangulated) resulting in a *cathartic* cure. *Breuer*'s theory for why the hysteric strangulated affect in the first place relied on a typical medical-model conception – that of the *hypnoid state*. This boils down to saying that certain persons are born with a proclivity to split consciousness, in what *Janet* (1920) had called a 'dissociation'.

That is, illness is postulated to develop from some unidirectional influence, presumably in the makeup of the genes, the blood, the structure of the brain, or whatever. Theories of this type flourish today, with a more modern variation adding the concept of genetic mutation. Just by chance one person has a crossing-over of chromosomal strains in mitosis, altering cellular structure in the subsequent course of physical development and bringing on the abnormal behavior witnessed at some point in life. This account is entirely efficient- and material-cause in nature (*Rychlak*, 1968, 1973). There is also the 'hint' of a formal-cause explanation here in that abnormal behavioral *patterns* can be diagnosed as syndromes of disease (hysteria versus schizophrenia, for example). But such patterns are themselves 'effects' of the underlying material and efficient causes, so the medical model holds that we must *reduce* the pattern to the substrate determinants in order to account for it.

Nowhere in this medical-model approach to abnormality are we to find a *final* cause explanation, a claim that behavior takes place 'for the sake of' some precedent intention, willful aspiration, self-directing desire, and so on. The energic 'powers' which run the body are reducible to chemical substrates where 'natural laws' of immutable determinisms function, moved along by anabolism and catabolism totally without a teleological purpose in view. Behavior flow is unidirectional, an input-output chain of events with memory storage influencing through habit what will occur. In the final analysis, there is no choice here – or at least, there is no role for choice in the development or manifestation of psychic disorder.

In his 1892 paper, *Freud* takes a different tack, altering this style of description in the medical model, and effectively reintroducing *teleological* factors into behavior. The prime case history described in this account is that of a young mother who had 'distressing symptoms' like vomiting, agitation, and loss of sleep when she was required to breast-feed her children. But there are several other examples cited of hysterical disorders, in which, though the individual would prefer to have one thing eventuate, an alternative behavior is brought about. For example, *Freud* tells of certain patients who see an improper, ugly or unusual behavior take place, and then *out of the fear* that they too might reproduce these behaviors actually *do* the improper thing. In one case it was reproducing the silly grimaces of a comedian.

Another form of this disorder seemed to arise when a school boy had a secret passion for a certain girl of his acquaintance. Keeping his secret proved difficult, but he managed until one day, while under a special excitement, he blurted out her name in the middle of a class. From that time onward into his adult years he retained this 'hysterical tic', calling forth 'Maria' from time to time. *Freud* also reported briefly on the case of Frau Emmy von N. in this paper, a patient who was to occupy a major portion of the Studies on Hysteria (*Breuer and Freud*, 1955, pp.48–105). In this case, Frau Emmy emitted a 'clacking' sound with her tongue which – *Freud* eventually determined via hypnosis – had begun one evening as she sat by the bedside of her young daughter, who was very ill, and said to herself 'Now you must be absolutely quiet, so as not to wake her' (*Freud*, 1966a, p. 124). The very next action was a pronounced 'clack' as if in direct opposition to the intended course of behavior (i. e., to be quiet).

Freud employed the constructs of a *counter-will* and *antithetic ideas* to account for hysterical disorders of this type. This theory suggested that human beings both intend to act in certain ways, and yet also hold certain expectations concerning the likelihood that they can actually put these intentions into effect. There is a subjective uncertainty in behavior, and with many if not all intentions we human beings generate immediate counter-intentions as 'antithetic ideas' to those intentions we really want to affirm and thereby reach 'motoric action' in behavior.

We can see in here the early glimmerings of *Freud*'s defense hypothesis, and what he will later call *repression*. But at this point in time, Freud cured this hapless young mother – whose distressing antithetical idea was probably something like 'I won't be able to breast-feed my children' – by aligning himself with the forces of the 'confident' intention. Putting his patient under a light hypnosis, *Freud* (1966a, p. 119) reassured her as follows: 'Have no fear! You will make an excellent nurse and the baby will thrive. Your stomach is perfectly quiet, your appetite is excellent, you are looking forward to your next meal, etc.' And, after only a few such treatments, the young woman was successfully brought back to maternal health. *Freud* had not yet put himself on the trail of the *reasons* or the *grounds* for the sake of which a 'I can't' or 'I won't' expectation was formulated in the personality structure. This was to come later, and it opened up a Pandora's box of sexual lust and hostility which was to alter the face of humanity for all time.

Anyone who reads *Freud* and who is aware of the historical bifurcation reviewed in Chapter 1 between the dialectical and the demonstrative form of theorizing must now be aware that *Freud* is a 20th Century dialectician trying to find his way within the strictures of a demonstrative science which does not quite meet his humanistic purposes. Freud's treatment has the individual forming intentions, and not only positive but also negative intentions, or, feared likelihoods that 'might' take place in direct opposition to what one wishes will be taking place. This dialectical premise alters our very thinking about behavior because now the options open to the behaving organism in the 'henceforth' are multiplied – at *least* by two: We have the possibility here of doing what we intend doing, or, in doing what we do *not* intend doing (what we 'fear' doing). There is also a burden put on the intellect here, a rumination about the future course of behavior which *cannot be avoided.*

Freud never explicated this side of his thinking, but what this treatment of behavior comes down to in a technical sense is the formulation of a teleological descriptive account. Though he would have preferred *not* to have relied on telic conceptions, there can be no doubt but that *Freud*'s image of man is purposive. One can see the working and reworking of his antithetical ideas theory throughout the 1890s period in *Freud*'s extended correspondence with *Wilhelm Fliess* (*Freud*, 1954). *Fliess*, whom *Freud* had met through the intercession of *Breuer*, was a nose and throat specialist with a very successful practice in Berlin. *Freud* seems to have used this contact as a continuing sounding board and source of support for his developing ideas during this very difficult but fruitful decade which *Freud* often remarked he lived through in 'splendid isolation' – including his self-analysis, the writing of his *Interpretation of Dreams* (*Freud*, 1953a), and the germination of all major psychoanalytical conceptions.

Freud suggests to *Fliess* that antithetical ideas were often the 'other side' of consciously stated intentions, precisely because the individual had initially toyed with them as his *true* attitude, wish, etc. (*Freud*, 1954, p. 147). The grounds affirmed, the position eventually taken, would constitute the 'that' in the 'that for the sake of which' phrasing of the final cause (see *Rychlak*, 1968, p. 231). Often these antithetical ideas were self-reproaches, self-denigrations motivated by a sense of guilt (itself, a judgment made of one's worth 'for the sake of' or on the basis of some principle). In 1896 he could say to *Fliess*: 'Indeed, it appears as though the whole psychical complex – recollection and self-reproach – is conscious at first. Later on, without anything fresh happening, both of them are repressed [the 'strangulation' concept of *Breuer*], and in their place an *antithetic symptom* is formed in consciousness' (*Freud*, 1954, p. 149). It would have been clearer if *Freud* had named the symptom a 'dialectical synthesis', for this is surely the meaning he conveyed – albeit unknowingly.

This is how it develops in psychoanalysis that a neurotic symptom is *always* a compromise formulation, representing symbolically the *repressing* wish and the *repressed* wish. The symptom as the dream is therefore always saying something. We can see directly in the symptom picture a manifestation of the underlying problem, if we but assume the proper (i. e., psychoanalytical) attitude in relation to it. For example, one of *Freud*'s female patients (Dora) suffered from a hysterical throat irritation which caused her to cough incessantly (*Freud*, 1953b). He traced this physical symptom to an unconscious fantasy in which this 19-year-old girl had thought of performing an act of fellatio, thanks in part to her oral propensities (oral fixations) and also in part to her oedipal desires for a penis of her own (actually for her father's penis; *Freud*, 1953b, pp. 47–48). The repressing attitude here (intention) is 'Sexual promptings like fellatio are both morally reprehensible and positively sickening' while at the same time a counter-will antithetical idea of 'I should like to perform fellatio' was dialectically defined. Result? In the clinical symptom of a sore throat and cough one finds both the partial realization of the antithetical idea (which might have been phantasized in a dream as actually taking place) *and* the socially 'proper' intentions of the young lady being realized (i. e., one is punished with illness, pain, 'a burden' and the like if she violates God's prescriptions).

The same kind of dialectical logic is to be seen in Freud's treatment of dreams as 'wish fulfillments'. The reason that some dreams are both wish-fulfilling and upsetting (nightmares, etc.) is because they like symptoms are invariably compromises. We have the id-prompting wish of, let us say, lascivious desires for a mother or mothersubstitute (male oedipal), but *also* the countering wish of the superego to contend with which promises dire outcomes for such unacceptable transgressions of the moral code. *Both* wishes are to be found compounded into a dream storyline, so it is *not* correct to say that dreams, which punish the dreamer, send him into a cold sweat out of fear, arouse him from slumber with 'the shakes', and so forth, contradict *Freud*'s hedonistic theories of behavior.

Freud's budding analytical insights of the 1890s burst into our awareness with a shock value – not so much for their sexualized content but for their dialectical quality. Even today, we ask: Could such business really be true? For example, *Freud* (1954, p. 273) says to *Fliess*:

> It turns out, for instance, that hysterical headaches are due to a fantastic parallel which equates the head with the other end of the body (hair in both places – cheeks and buttocks – lips and labiae – mouth and vagina); so that a migraine can be used to represent a forcible defloration, the illness thus again standing for a wish-fulfillment.

The migraine patient could have her psychic cake and eat it too. Her repressed wish (antithetical ideas, to be seduced or raped) might be accomplished 'symbolically' (or in a dream) even as the repressing wish for punishment (intention: propriety demands punishment for impropriety) could be satisfied as well.

Freud thus evolved a model of illness in which the personality structure sought a certain adjustment level, with the ego as the 'man in the middle' seeking a balance between the unacceptable intentions (wishes, originally antithetical ideas) of the id and the socially more appropriate intentions (wishes) of the *ego* and *superego* (*Freud* occasionally used the latter concepts interchangeably). The writer has heard supposed criticisms of *Freud* based on the 'weakness' of having to reduce the 'one person' into 'three, little people' as is done in the id, ego, and superego conceptualizations. But this 'one in many' dialectical formulation is perfectly understandable and historically precedented in countless theories as surveyed in Chapter 1 of the present volume. It seems illogical to break the human person up this way only if one is reasoning demonstratively. This made illness an assessment of the adequacy of personality functioning, an idea which was quite foreign to the efficiently caused mechanistic theories like those of *Breuer* and *Janet*. It was not illness which thereby acquired a final cause, not disease which gained a mentality, but rather the man, or the 'personality', about whom a judgment of mental normality was being made.

There is a certain irony in the fact that a man who began his conceptualizations entirely at the level of intentional analysis, and who on more than one occasion challenged *Fliess* to suggest how they might in some way explain things 'physiologically' or 'organically' (*Freud*, 1954, pp. 169, 265), was to end up as apostle for instinctive drives and mental energies. Yet anyone who takes a detailed look at his libido theory must surely appreciate that this is a superficial theoretical device, a move on the part of *Freud* to retain the 'sound' of classical medical theory, even as he was changing the model in dramatic fashion (*Rychlak*, 1968, 1973). From his very first fumbling attempts to describe behavior in terms of mental energies (see e. g. F., *Freud*, 1962, pp. 60–61), *Freud* reaches for something other than exclusively material- and efficient-cause meanings. There would be nothing uniquely Freudian in viewing mental energies as forces which propel the organism when they rise and cease this propulsion as they fall off in volume or level. The blind hedonism of a 'rat psychologist' makes use of such concepts and we do not think of these theories as in any way like *Freud*'s.

What then *is* peculiar to *Freud*'s mental energies? The fact that in his theoretical formulations *drive power* always issued from a dialectical ploy of some sort, oriented teleologically for some goal, and then rephrased in energy terms after the implications were clear. It was not merely the instinctual drive or its (efficient-cause) 'energy' which provided the dynamics of motion, but the energy as stimulated and then opposed by another, oppositional (antithetical) 'energy' which called for a resolution or synthesis in repression, projection, sublimation, or whatever. Energies which run to their expenditure in physics are never manipulated with 'strategies' (formal causes) 'for the sake of which' (final causes) one side of the mind (id) makes itself known through a devious parapraxis despite the vigilance of an opposing side of mind (ego, superego). In the Freudian unconscious there *is* trickery and deceit, ploy and counterploy, until one's head is sent spinning trying to keep up with the machinations supposedly going on. Each client is a marvel of intricate detail and fascinating motivation.

In short, an honest appraisal can only suggest that *Freud* made his energies (a) behave dialectically and (b) carry out intentions, including compromises therein. That he was not entirely without appreciation of the fact that the libido theory was 'tacked on' to his image of man is gleaned in the following comment, made in 1914: 'I should like at this point expressly to admit that the hypothesis of separate ego-instincts and sexual instincts (that is to say, the libido theory) rests scarcely at all upon a psychological basis, but derives its principal support from biology" (*Freud*, 1957 a, p. 79). The truth is, *Freud* could always explain the same mental dynamic in a psychoanalytical fashion with *or* without a libidinal phrasing.

If *Freud* did not need an energy concept, but merely brought this in out of deference to his colleagues and the pressures of friends, how then could he arrive at an image of *psychic determinism*? Is not the concept of determinism possible only when based upon an energy concept? Actually, determinism and final causation are not mutually contradictory conceptions. In fact, historically, hard determinism (rigidly predictable events) began in the assumptions of a 'perfect universe' as created by the *intentional* design of a God (deity teleology). Even in the pre-Christian hard-determinism theories of *Democritus*, the idea that 'nothing happens by chance' was buttressed by the corollary notion that there is a 'rationale' (formal-cause pattern) 'for the sake of which' (final cause) Nature (as construed by God) is continually functioning. To speak of chance is thus to err due to ignorance of the rationale behind events (*Magill and McGreal*, 1961, p. 40). If we now take a comparable approach to Freudian theory, and consider it a final-cause theory of mentality (a *human* teleology), then psychic determinism can be seen as the 'weight of logic' or the 'necessity of reason'. Though the brain may 'work' by exchanges of a physical energy and the motions of physical atoms in the cell membranes (efficient and material causation) – as does any body in general – the pressure of logical necessity (formal-final causation) may be what determines which ideas will be carried over into action, repressed, or fended off into a compromise solution of some sort.

Freud was drawn to this very tactic of using what some have called 'emotional syllogisms', as when he discussed paranoid projection developing from a proposition of the sort '*I* (a man) *love him* (a man)' (*Freud*, 1958, p. 63). If we now provide the backdrop major premise here of 'All homosexuals are mad' or 'Only a filthy, degenerate subhuman could love a member of his own sex', we can see the *necessary* conclusion to follow if a man now senses 'I love him'. The implication, the flow of reasoning as *Aristotle* has taught us (refer to Chapter 1), moves from premises to conclusions. The import is there without alternative *if* we really *do believe* the backdrop assumptions. Ideas having this import are naturally avoided by the individual, or conclusions of this sort may not be drawn consciously. In fact, the individual may keep from aligning such premises to a conclusion through all manner of Freudian defensive maneuvers. Yet the *necessary* aspects of this line of reasoning fall into order ('that for the sake of which' we believe) once the proper premises have been patterned (formal cause). The necessity does not come secondarily into play, thanks so the 'pressure' of a mental energy on the hydraulic analogy of steam-driving a piston.

There are some concrete examples in his writings where *Freud* dealt with what are clearly dialectical issues. In 1910, some 18 years after his antithetic-ideas paper, *Freud* (1957b) returned to this topic in a work entitled 'The Antithetical Meaning of Primal Words'. The text was based upon the work of the philologist *Karl Abel*, and it delighted *Freud* for *Abel* had evidence to suggest that in the earliest known examples of human languages, such as Egyptian, 'there are a fair number of words with two meanings, one of which is the exact opposite of the other' (*Freud*, 1957b, p. 156). *Abel* contended that man's earliest mental concepts emerged as an undifferentiated total (one in many), which subsumed opposites, and only by guessing from context could one person understand what another person was referring to. Thus, the concept of strength doubtless first expressed the contrary ideas of strong versus weak. It was this relationship between opposite meanings that man first captured in language as a single term. It was important for *Freud* to have such views at his elbow, because many of his critics found his twists and turns as theoretician to be excessive.

Freud also liked to use a writing style in his longer papers which took on a Socratic, dialectical tone. That is, he presented his case to an imaginary opponent who countered with questions and challenges in opposition to his contentions (see, e. g., *Freud*, 1961, p. 21). In fact, *Freud*'s basic writing style has this polemical feature throughout, in which he often raises objections 'for the reader' before carrying on his line of thought. This brings the reader into the evolving point of view, almost as if a dialogue were in progress.

Even so, *Freud* was unaware of the intellectual tradition within which he theorized, and he would in fact have rejected the 'appellation' of dialectician. He equated dialectic with sophistry or senseless argumentation, motivated more by personal than scientific reasons. He makes this attitude clear in the following: 'I have never been able to convince myself of the truth of the maxim that strife is the father of all things. I believe it is derived from the Greek sophists and is at fault, like them, through overvaluing dialectics' (*Freud*, 1963, pp. 244–245). These are strange words from a man who fought the resistance of the censor, broke with most of his former mentors and students, said of himself that he always needed an enemy to oppose as well as a close friend in whom to confide, stood against a generation of his fellow scientists confident in the belief that they were too threatened or constricted by their own sexual repressions to look objectively at the truth, and who spent the larger part of his life in dialectical exchanges with patients, colleagues, students, and the readers of his books.

Only *Freud*, the man who could give the most banal acts an oppositional twist to set one's head spinning, could also in 1937 dismiss the dialectic with a cool sentence in a letter to *R. L. Worrall* concerning Marxian theory: 'As to the "dialectic", I am no clearer, even after your letter' (*Jones*, 1957, p. 345). Since *Freud* viewed dialectical analysis as sophistry, could it be that he did not wish to find the obvious parallels between his 'method' and this classical organon? We must give this point serious consideration, for there is no doubt but that *Freud*'s concept of psychoanalysis was more as a scientific method than as a method of therapy (see *Rychlak*, 1973, pp. 225–226). Of course, *Freud* (as *Hegel* and *Marx* before him) made only selective use of dialectical formulations. A more sagacious dialectician could have accepted the fact that more than one view of the case history might have eventuated in cures. This is what history was to teach, for *Adler*, *Jung*, and *Rank* all garnered their quota of cures based upon somewhat different premises of human nature. And when *Freud* had to confront these alternative formulations, there was no way in which to resolve the issue – without moving to the laboratory form of experiment. But that was never to be. Instead, we witness a falling out, a leaving the parental group, and an establishing of alternative 'schools' of psychoanalysis in the Adlerian, Jungian, and Rankian variations.

But even these schools have retained in large measure the spirit of dialectic. To cure mental disease *Freud* found it necessary (a) first to identify the premises, or 'prototypical' imagos (formal causes) which presaged the illness and thus logically determined that it be expressed (as per our review of psychic determinism, above); (b) through dialectical examination, turn the patient back on his unnamed or unknown (unconscious) premises and see the 'why' of his current behavior (the 'that for the sake of which' he behaves); and then (c) help establish an alternative set of premises on which to behave (a different 'one' within the many possible). The Democritan rationale had been changed in some way and hence it *necessarily* (psychic determinism) altered the way in which life was to be patterned in the henceforth. We find the same strategy in Adlerian (*Adler*,

1964) therapy where prototypical life styles must be fully described to the individual in order that he may change his (usually selfish) way of behaving. *Jung* (1954) asks that we base psychology on a teleological principle, and that the mentally sick individual recognize a (patterned) side of his psyche which he 'is not', and thereby balance off the four points of his psychic compass. *Rank* (1945) conceived of the therapeutic relationship as a (dialectical) confrontation – a 'battle', actually – in which the resultant contradictions between therapist and client had to be resolved in favor of the latter if a cure was to eventuate.

It was this dialectical heritage which *Freud actually* left the field of psychopathology, even though he was to confound it with pseudobiological explanations. In time, *Freud* came to talk more in terms of this physicalistic lingo, but it is clear that he never thought about human behavior in these demonstrative, efficient-cause terms. His one effort to do so, the ill-fated 'project for a scientific psychology' (*Freud,* 1966b), which he began under the incessant prodding of *Fliess*, was never completed and *Freud* later tried to have it destroyed as simply not reflective of his thought. *Freud* was a great albeit reluctant and selective dialectician (i. e., he could not brook alternatives to his view by colleagues). We must place his genius in proper historical perspective, and take from it that which is most valuable to our understanding of the human situation. Freudian psychology is *impossible* without its dialectical foundations.

References

Adler, A.: Problems of neurosis (Harper & Row, New York 1964).

Breuer, J. and Freud, S.: On the psychical mechanism of hysterical phenomena: preliminary communication; in *Strachey* The standard edition of the complete psychological works of Sigmund Freud, vol. II, pp. 1–17 (Hogarth Press, London 1955).

Freud, S.: The interpretation of dreams; in *Strachey* The standard edition of the complete psychological works of Sigmund Freud, vol. IV, V (Hogarth, London 1953a).

Freud, S.: Fragment of an analysis of a case of hysteria; in *Strachey* The standard edition of the complete psychological works of Sigmund Freud vol. VII, pp. 3–112 (Hogarth, London 1953b).

Freud, S.: The origins of psycho-analysis: letters to Wilhelm Fliess, drafts and notes: 1887–1902 (Basic Books, New York 1954).

Freud, S.: On narcissism: an introduction; in *Strachey* The standard edition of the complete psychological works of Sigmund Freud, vol. XIV, pp. 67–102 (Hogarth, London 1957a).

Freud, S.: The antithetical meaning of primal words; in *Strachey* The standard edition of the complete psychological works of Sigmund Freud, vol. XI, pp. 153–162 (Hogarth, London 1957b).

Freud, S.: Psycho-analytic notes on an autobiographical account of a case of paranoia; in *Strachey* The standard edition of the complete psychological works of Sigmund Freud, vol. XII, pp. 1–82 (Hogarth, London 1958).

Freud, S.: The future of an illusion; in *Strachey* The standard edition of the complete psychological works of Sigmund Freud, vol. XXI, pp. 1–56 (Hogarth, London 1961).

Freud, S.: The neuro-psychoses of defence; in *Strachey* The standard edition of the complete psychological works of Sigmund Freud, vol. III, pp. 45–61 (Hogarth, London 1962).

Freud, S.: Introductory lectures on psycho-analysis. Part III; in *Strachey* The standard edition of the complete psychological works of Sigmund Freud, vol. XVI (Hogarth, London 1963).

Freud, S.: A case of successful treatment by hypnotism; in *Strachey* The standard edition of the complete psychological works of Sigmund Freud, vol. I, pp. 115–128 (Hogarth, London 1966a).

Freud, S.: Project for a scientific psychology; in *Strachey* The standard edition of the complete psychological works of Sigmund Freud, vol. I, pp. 281–397 (Hogarth, London 1966b).

Janet, P.: The major symptoms of hysteria; 2nd. ed. (Macmillan, New York, 1920).

Jones, E.: The life and work of Sigmund Freud: the last phase, vol. 3 (Basic Books, New York 1957).

Jung, C. G.: The practice of psychotherapy, in *Read, Fordham and Adler* The collected works of C. G. Jung, vol. 16. Bollingen Series XX.16 (Pantheon Books / Routledge & Kegan, New York / London, 1954).

Magill, F. N. and McGreal, I. P.: Masterpieces of world philosophy, vol. I, II (Salem Press, New York 1961).

Rank, O.: Will therapy, and truth and reality (Knopf, New York 1945).

Rychlak, J. F.: A philosophy of science for personality theory (Houghton Mifflin, Boston 1968).

Rychlak, J. F.: Introduction to personality and psychotherapy: a theory-construction approach (Houghton Mifflin, Boston 1973).

Contr. hum. Dev., vol. 2, pp. 44–52 (Karger, Basel 1976)

Chapter 5
Male and Female: The Search for Synthesis

Nancy Datan

Introduction

This chapter explores dimensions of belief and disbelief in, of and between the sexes. Its central thesis is a dialectical model of sexuality, a model in which thesis and antithesis arise out of the same source, the psychoanalytic model of development. I shall suggest that somewhere inside each of us is the 7-year-old who cannot believe that the basis for sexual differentiation admits of a reductionist explanation, whether it is genetic or cultural. I will argue that the woman in a bikini, the woman in labour, the man at a plow, or coming up to bat in the World Series, cannot be explained simply through recourse to biology nor by an appeal to established, functional sex roles. I shall propose that the behaviors which comprise sex roles do not provide a basis for differentiation between the sexes; that, indeed, sex-role differentiation arises out of an impulse within the individual to differentiate himself or herself relative to the other – to his sexual opposite. In this way the sexes define each other: sex roles do not serve merely as a convenient division of the tasks necessary to the survival of the individual and the species, nor do they demonstrate any mandatory tie to the biological imperatives of reproduction.

As *Mead*'s (1949) studies of sex and temperament indicate, some form of sex-role differentiation can be expected in most cultures, but the form of this differentiation does not inevitably reflect the temporary passivity of the woman during pregnancy and childbearing. While the dominant male and the submissive female are easily called to mind as sex-role stereotypes, the nurturant female and the male seeking sanctuary with her are also readily recognized. Sex-role differentiation, then, is not defined as any fixed set of behaviors which are invariably male or female, but rather expressed by a polarity in behavior, one sex defining the other and defined by it.

I consider that what is seen at 7 as an arbitrary imposition of one sex or the other upon an individual who was originally dual – a view first voiced by *Plato*, and more recently expressed by *Freud* – becomes at 17 a sexual identity which is eagerly affirmed in the presence of the opposite sexual identity. More briefly, I shall suggest that although the explanation of the ontological necessity for sexual differentiation is lost somewhere in the evolution of our species, current manifestations of this differentiation – ranging from traditional sex roles to the ebb and flow of feminist movements – do not derive directly from biology, and cannot be explained by functional sociological analysis. The origin of these differing behaviors, I shall propose, is more plausibly traced to the mating dance, to ritual courtship behavior in which any act is defined by its effect upon the partner. Thus, the sexes not only define, but create and affirm, one another, in an ongoing dialectic of behavior.

The Unconscious Dialectic: Theoretical Antecedents and Current Status

Plato (1952) wrote in the *Symposium* that people were originally bisexual, and that the gods, jealous of the joy of union, divided each one into two: and, subsequently, the world has been a place of half-persons seeking their other halves. *Freud* (1933) has described this duality of nature as unitary in expression: that is, his essay on femininity stressed the bisexual nature of man and woman. He argued that there were dynamic components of personality in each sex which reflected both so-called masculine and so-called feminine traits. The distinction between the sexes, he maintained, was more complex and more profound than a stereotyped sex role: the equating of active with masculine, for example, failed to acknowledge the active nature of the mother's interaction with her child, as well as overlooking species in which females were the stronger and the more aggressive. His tentative conclusion was that constitutional determinants and social customs interacted to produce women who, in the main, might be described as having passive aims (in the service of which they might be very active), and men whose aims might be described as active. Masculine and feminine traits could be seen in both men and women.

This temperate statement, with its emphasis upon the complexity of determinants of 'masculinity' and 'femininity', its assertion of bisexuality in both men and women, and its argument against the equation of passivity with femininity, activity with masculinity, is not the statement generally associated with *Freud*'s views on women. *Freud* (1933, p. 124) is better known among feminists for his insistence – in the latter half of his essay on femininity which begins so temperately – upon the universality of penis envy among women, and for his declaration that 'the anatomical distinction between the sexes must express itself in psychical consequences'.

This paper takes *Freud*'s declaration as its point of departure, and in doing so, restates the banal. Humans are born small and helpless, and remain small and dependent longer than other animals do: 'It is human to have a long childhood', remarks *Erikson* (1963, p. 16); 'it is civilised to have an ever longer childhood.' It is our destiny, then, to 'look up' to those in power, since when their power is greatest, they are large and we are little.

We are also born male or female, and so, at birth, our role in the act of reproduction is determined: either we sire children, and do not know what it is like to bear them, or we bear children, and do not know what it is like to sire them. The very rare exceptions – such as transsexual surgery – do not blur the boundaries between the sexes, but rather stress the desires of the majority to discover – at least vicariously, through reports – what it is like to have been both male and female.

Bettelheim (1962) has further explored *Freud*'s assertion that anatomy is destiny, and, while his work with schizophrenic children has supported *Freud*'s controversial view of a widespread penis envy among women, he has found that this is only one half of the dynamic relationship between the sexes. Across a variety of primitive cultures, *Bettelheim* found support for a complementary envy which he first observed among the boys at the Orthogenic School: womb envy, manifest in adolescent rituals which, through mutilation of the genitals, mimics the bleeding – and assurance of sexual maturity – which is woman's at menarche. *Bettelheim* goes on to suggest that although there is in each sex a measure of envy, neither sex wishes to possess the characteristics of the other at the expense of what is already theirs: that is, neither in penis envy nor in womb envy is there a desire to relinquish one's own sex, but merely the desire for additional acquisition: to have not one sex, nor the other, but both.

Bettelheim's model, like the less complete Freudian model of penis envy, is reminiscent of the Platonic legend of the 'complete' person, who unites both sexes in one body. *Freud* and *Bettelheim* imply an unconscious dialectical relationship between the sexes, of ongoing incomplete efforts by each at possession of the powers of the other. As *Plato*'s legend indicates, these efforts find a partially successful expression through heterosexual union, evocatively described by *Freud* (1963, p. 13):

> At the height of being in love the boundary between ego and object threatens to melt away. Against all the evidence of his senses, a man who is in love declares that 'I' and 'you' are one, and is prepared to behave as if it were a fact.

Heterosexual love does not, however, resolve the conflicting desires of the sexes to possess one another's attributes. On the contrary, sexual union throughout human history has introduced a new dimension into the dialectical conflict between the sexes. Where there were two adults, whose sexual natures were complementary and who, in other respects, were similar, sexual union creates a third participant. Unborn, this third is parasitic upon the body of the female causing her to be temporarily somewhat dependent upon the male; and, when born, this third individual introduces into a union of two adults a new set of needs.

The Parental Imperative: A Situational Dialectic

The paradox of sexual union bears some reconsideration and review. Two adults, a man and a woman, seek union with one another; and out of that union comes a third small person who, according to psychoanalytic models of development, is engaged in another dimension of dialectical conflict, seeking to regain a union lost at birth (*Erikson*, 1963). The parental relationship to this small person, if successful, is a dialectic of nurturance and dependency. And out of this relationship comes a further paradox; i. e., if parental nurturance is successful, the dependent infant grows into the independent young adult and outgrows the need for parental care.

The psychoanalytic view of sexuality postulates the existence of 'male' and 'female' characteristics in both sexes. Nevertheless, in most cultures, for most of human history, child care has been the domain of women, while men's tasks have taken them into the field, the forest, or the office, to pursue more 'aggressive' activities. *Gutmann* (1973, 1975) has suggested that the near-universal sex-role division, in which mother is nurturant and minds the home and father aggressively secures a living for the family, is not a consequence of innate differences in disposition, but rather a response to the presence of a child. *Gutmann* characterizes the period of parenthood as one of 'chronic emergency' for which the most effective coping strategy is a division of roles in which the woman surrenders to her husband, as it were, her aggressive potential, while he surrenders to his wife his need for nurturance and passivity. This role division is achieved despite an underlying constitutional similarity of the parents. The child's needs are met by the nurturant mother; and the needs of the mother and child for shelter and protection are met by the aggressive father.

The original dialectic between male and female, adult individuals with comparable natures complicated by unconscious desires to possess not only their own sex but the characteristics of the opposite sex as well, has created new dimensions of dialectic: i. e., between the narcissistic, dependant infant and nurturant mother, and, between the dependent mother-child and the providing father. The successful outcome of these dialectical dependencies is an independent young adult; indeed, any parent-child relationship which prolongs dependency is pathological. And so the dialectic between parent and child contains within itself its own obsolescence, with implications for sex-role changes in women and men whose children have attained independence.

The Changes of Middle Age: Dialectic Over the Life Cycle

Studies of personality change based on projective responses over the life cycle among subjects of various ages have indicated that the stereotyped masculine and feminine traits are reversed in middle age; that is, women repossess a measure of their innate aggression, manifest as managerial, domineering behavior, while men become more nurturant and passive (*Gutmann*, 1964; *Neugarten and Gutmann*, 1958). *Gutmann* (1975) has suggested that the onset of middle age, and the intrapsychic shifts seen in projective responses, reflect the ebbing of the 'chronic emergency' of parenthood. He called this phase of the life cycle the 'normal unisex of later life'. In the absence of urgent demands by children during later life, which was the stimulus which precipitated the sex-role division of young adulthood, the original bisexual nature of each partner finds greater freedom for expression resulting in a relative reversal of 'masculine' and 'feminine' traits.

The intrapsychic changes, which are shown to be bound up with the family life cycle, are consistent with external changes in the lifelines of men and women. For men, this is a period of career peak and then plateau or decline; for women, middle age may be a time to enter or to return to the labor force (*Neugarten and Moore*, 1968); for middle class men, this period of the life cycle may be seen as one of job boredom, while women sense a new phase of the life cycle opening up for them (*Neugarten*, 1968).

The life cycle, then, reflects a succession of dialectical transformations in adulthood which grow out of a succession of paradoxes. A man and a woman, in seeking union, create a child, which causes them to take on sex-typed roles; the child is cared for, grows to adulthood and independence, and the parents' sex-typed roles – the dialectic of parenthood – become unnecessary, and, indeed, so far as the child is concerned, irrelevant. In middle age, then, the poles are reversed, and women assume the dominance which was men's, while men permit themselves the passivity which was – seemingly – the prerogative of women earlier in the life cycle.

Revolution and Reaction: Dialectic in Feminism

The sex-role division described here as the normative response to the 'chronic emergency' of parenthood has come under attack in recent years by feminists, who argue that it is possible for women to enjoy the fruits of conquest and achievement, and for men to enjoy their own nurturance, earlier in the life cycle, through a more egalitarian sharing of roles, that is to say, by the elimination of what has been described here as the dialectic of parenthood. It is not my purpose to enter this controversy, but rather to review past controversies, and, on the basis of this review, offer some observations which set the controversies of feminism into the context of the unconscious dialectic described in psychoanalytic theory.

The goals of modern feminism are not new. A comparable movement for equal economic, political, and social status for women took place in Central Europe over a century ago (*Datan*, 1972), and a similar movement occurred in the United States at the start of the present century (*Datan*, 1973). Both movements were followed by what feminists have viewed as a regression to tradition, in which, despite steps toward egalitarianism such as the enactment of a law giving women the vote, there was a movement among women away from strong career involvement and in the direction of the domestic role.

I do not intend to ask why feminism has failed – if it has failed – in the past, nor to speculate on its future. It seems to me that there is another question worth asking, a question which, if answered, may yield insight into the rhythm of revolution and reaction in feminism: Why is there no masculinism movement? This question has not been explored, for its answer has seemed apparent: men command high status, men have nothing to gain by a reexamination of traditional roles. Women do have something to gain, through an expansion of their available options. Men have no real additional options available to them reflecting achievement: the apparent option of increased involvement in child care requires a partial relinquishment of career achievement in the service of a nurturant role which – at least at the start of the child's life, when the parental role is most vital – cannot be as completely involving as the woman's role. Anatomy permits the woman a destiny in which she bears and suckles a child; feminism allows her a career as well: the most nurturant of fathers can only give his child a bottle, not his body. The modification of traditional roles for women and men in the direction of 'liberation', then can be interpreted as leading to an increment for women, a decrement for men.

The possibility of a narrowed range of options for men – at least relative to the expanded options avaiable to women – would serve to explain hostility among men toward feminist movements, and there is, indeed evidence of this hostility. Moreover, I have argued (*Datan*, 1975) that this hostility has ancient roots: the antagonism between female procreativity and male creativity can be traced, in the history of Western civilization, to pre-Mosaic fertility religions, which were not only displaced by Judaism and later by Christianity, but were repeatedly proscribed. As *Freud* and others have observed, the most effective way to discover our strongest urges is through the study of law: if an action were not powerfully tempting, it would hardly be necessary to forbid it. Furthermore, I have suggested that the cyclical rhythm of orgy and mourning of the Canaanites has not, in fact, disappeared, but has been incorporated, in muted and civilized form, into the holidays of Judaism and Christianity (*Datan*, 1975), and, finally, I have noted that the move away from the propitiation of nature gods accompanied other dimensions of civilization which reflected mastery by man over nature. The Goddess of the Canaanites was usurped by the God of the Jews, and her procreativity was usurped, finally, by the Immaculate Conception of Christianity; yet no woman today would exchange the relatively subordinate status of women in Judaeo-Christian tradition for the hazards of procreation 5,000 years ago which led men to worship the Goddess of birth and death.

There is historical support, then, for the feminist perception of hostility among men toward changes in women's roles. I would argue, however, that this hostility is only marginally related to changes in the status differential between men and women, and that its basis is in men's recognition of the existential limits of sex. Procreativity, and primary involvement with the infant when his needs are greatest, are the domain of women, and are not accessible to men; while the sublimated creativity which is typically the domain of men can be, and has been, available to women.

I do not think it is possible, however, to move from a recognition of men's antagonism to the women's movement to the assertion that it is this antagonism which has obstructed the steady progress of women toward a more egalitarian position in contemporary society. Revolution in women's roles has occurred despite some male antagonism, and quite often, as in the case of the broad-scale revolution in sex roles on the Israeli kibbutz, has involved strong cooperative efforts by men. The history of women's movements does not bear out the view that men have prevented the progress of women toward equal status. And so it is reasonable to conclude, if revolutionary efforts to achieve equality between the sexes in Europe, Asia, and America have been followed by apparent regressions to tradition, the traditional role must be exercising an appeal for women which has generally been overlooked (*Datan*, 1972, 1973).

I have elsewhere described sex-role differentiation in two very different cultures, a kibbutz and a Muslim Arab village, which occupy two very similar ecological niches (*Datan*, in press); and I have shown that in each case, sex-role differentiation can be seen to be adaptive: cultural patterns are fitted to the enviroment. A broad-scale investigation of women in five Israeli subcultures ranging along a continuum from traditionalism to modernity, carried out by *Aaron Antonovsky*, *Benjamin Maoz*, and myself, indicated that psychological well-being was highest at the two extremes. While our data do not permit a conclusive study of the cultural determinants of well-being, I have suggested (*Datan*, 1972) that both traditional and modern cultures provide women with an opportunity for active achievement, although the nature of the achievement is, of course, different in the two cultural settings.

I think it is possible to suggest that if men are antagonistic to the new options available for women, women may be ambivalent; with tradition comes certainty; modernity brings options, and the necessity for choice. Our study suggests that the traditional role may persist because of an enduring appeal which it exerts for women; and, it is and has been possible for women to reject all components of the traditional role, including childbearing. If men are sometimes antagonistic to the expansion of women's options when no comparable expansion is available to them, it is also reasonable to interpret the recurrent 'regression' to traditional roles by women as the outcome of an examination of these options, and, in some cases, a resultant choice of the traditional role.

Male and Female: The Inevitability of Synthesis

There is no mandate for tradition. There is not only considerable variability in sex roles, but it is also possible to reject the traditional sex roles altogether, and to repudiate sexual union and reproduction. Most cultures allow for a measure of deviance, and some, like traditional Catholicism, have sanctioned celibacy; others, like the ancient Greeks, have sanctioned homosexuality. Of course, cultures in which sexual reproduction is not the norm become extinct; therefore, our historical and genetic inheritance predisposes us toward heterosexual union and reproduction. Social and genetic characteristics which – though they may enrich the life of the individual – do not lead to reproduction, whether planned or accidental, are characteristics which are not carried forward to the next generation. The outcome of this continual process of selection is a collection of individuals constitutionally inclined to heterosexual reproduction and cultural patterns which must therefore favor reproduction. And, with the added dimension of centuries of evolution, one can see the truth of *Freud*'s claim that 'anatomy is destiny', interpreting anatomy broadly to include not only a predetermined sex and thus a prescribed role in reproduction, but also an inherited drive to reproduce. In this sense, a measure of synthesis between male and female is, if not inevitable, certainly highly probable.

The sexual dialectic, then, is the outcome of innately bisexual constitutions which must find expression within the existential boundaries of sex and time. A man cannot achieve the procreativity of pregnancy and birth; a woman who seeks the sublimated creativity of men must do so at the expense of time which could otherwise be given over to children. Studies of unconscious dynamics, role change over the life cycle, and changes in women's roles seem to suggest that it is human nature to assert our own sexuality and to seek to possess the prerogatives of the opposite sex: while we may achieve partial resolution of one or another components of these conflicting needs, it is our fate to achieve no more than incomplete success.

References

Bettelheim, B.: Symbolic wounds; rev. ed. (Collier, New York 1962).

Datan, N.: To be a woman in Israel. Sch. Rev. *80:* 319–332 (1972).

Datan, N.: Your daughters shall prophesy: ancient and contemporary perspectives on the women of Israel; in *Curtis and Chertoff* Israel: Social structure and change (Transaction Books, New Brunswick 1973).

Datan, N.: Astarte, Moses, and Mary: perspectives on the sexual dialectic in Canaanite, Judaic, and Christian tradition; in *Riegel and Meacham* The developing individual in a changing world, vol. I (Mouton, The Hague 1975).

Datan, N.: Ecological antecedents and sex role consequences in traditional and modern Israeli sub-cultures; in *Schlegel* Emergent women (University of Pittsburgh Press, Pittsburgh, in press).

Erikson, E. H.: Childhood and society; rev. ed. (Norton, New York 1963).

Freud, S.: New introductory lectures on psychoanalysis (Norton, New York 1933).

Freud, S.: Civilization and its discontents (Norton, New York 1961).

Gutmann, D.: An exploration of ego configurations in middle and later life; in *Neugarten et al.* Personality in middle and late life (Atherton, New York 1964).

Gutmann, D.: Men, women, and the parental imperative. Commentary. December 1973.

Gutmann, D.: Parenthood: key to the comparative study of the life cycle; in *Datan and Ginsberg* Life-span developmental psychology: normative life crises (Academic Press, New York 1975).

Mead, M.: Male and female (Morrow, New York 1949).

Neugarten, B. L.: The awareness of middle age; in *Neugarten* Middle age and aging (University of Chicago Press, Chicago 1968).

Neugarten, B. L. and Gutmann, D.: Age-sex roles and personality in middle age: a thematic apperception study. Psychol. Monogr. *72:* No. 17, whole No. 470 (1958).

Neugarten, B. L. and Moore, J. W.: The changing age-status system; in *Neugarten* Middle age and aging (The University of Chicago Press, Chicago 1968).

Plato: Symposium; in *Hutchins* Great books of the western world, pp. 149–173 (Encyclopedia Britannica, Chicago 1952).

Contr. hum. Dev., vol. 2, pp 53–59 (Karger, Basel 1976)

Chapter 6
Dialectical Aspects of Moral Development

Robert Hogan

The present chapter explores the utility of the dialectical perspective as a means for understanding moral conduct and development. As the term is used here, the dialectic characterizes a particular way of thinking about the world, a viewpoint which *Pepper* (1942) called *organicism*. Organicism can be best understood by comparing it with positivism, the metaphysics of much contemporary social science. Positivism validates statements about the world through a process known as social verification in accordance with a correspondence theory of truth. Social verification consists of the repetition or successive validation of the same fact by one or several observers, and the persuasive force of such validation comes from the number of observations made of that fact, and the number of people who agree about it – thus the persuasive force is social. The correspondence theory of truth holds that a hypothesis is true if it leads to a successful prediction; truth is equated with verification, with the relationship between a hypothesis and its outcome. In the correspondence theory of truth, a true statement provides no insight into the underlying nature of reality; it merely specifies a repeatable observation – we know what goes with what but we never know why.

Organicism contrasts with positivism at virtually every point. Organicism validates statements about the world through a process known as constructive verification in accordance with a coherence theory of truth. Constructive verification consists of marshalling an array of different facts, taken from a variety of sources, that should converge to establish a single point. The persuasive force of constructive verification depends on the number of different facts that can be brought to bear on a proposition and their interrelationships. Consequently, this form of verification is more individual than social; the investigator must have sufficient imagination and intelligence to formulate a proposition that ties together a body of diverse facts and to show that the various facts are indeed related. Constructed data never exist in isolation; rather, each item of evidence is qualified by its relationship to all the other relevant data. Thus, there are no pure facts; all facts must be interpreted. According to the coherence theory of truth, the more true a proposition, the more closely will the facts that it encompasses be related and the more facts will it organize and bring together. The dialectic may be defined (at least for the social sciences) as a way of thinking about problems that emphasizes naturalistic observations and the analytical skill of the investigator and that takes account of the interrelated yet contradictory nature of experience (see Chapter 10); it is an intellectual style that searches for critical paradoxes, polarities, or discontinuities in nature and then attempts to reconcile them in terms of more fundamental principles. The dialectic is the thought form or intellectual style that characterizes organicism; yet, although every organicist thinks dialectically, not everyone who uses the dialectic is an organicist.

Now that we have defined dialectical thought we must describe the developmental perspective. Once this is done, the role of the dialectic in conceptions of moral development should be obvious. Two themes define the developmental perspective. The first is that there are natural endpoints to development, endpoints that are reached by qualitative changes over time. The second theme is that life is a continuous process of adjusting internal conditions to external demands, and these adjustments are made necessary by changes that occur in both the organism and the environment. With these criteria in mind, two points about developmental psychology become clear. First, organicism, with its emphasis on the interrelatedness of hypothesis and data and on the discontinuities in the development of knowledge, can be seen as a formal or very general statement of the developmental perspective. Thus, the dialectical mode of thought seems to be common to both organicism and developmental theory. Second, behaviorist-inspired theories of development, such, for example, as that provided by *Bandura* (1969), are not, properly speaking, developmental. In the social learning view there are no natural goals to development, nor do the dynamics of children's behavior undergo qualitative changes over time. Rather the child accumulates responses in a monotonic fashion in accordance with the goals defined by his caretakers, and the point at which growth and change stops is arbitrary.

In contrast with most American behaviorists, many Europeans and cognitive psychologists employ the dialectical perspective and are, consequently, more truly developmental in their viewpoints. Let us turn to a brief review of three very influential models of moral development (i. e., those provided by *Freud, Mead,* and *Piaget*). This review should show that, although all three refelct the dialectic, each is also inadequate when considered from a dialectical perspective.

The Psychoanalytic Model

Freud's dim view of man's nature caused him to see the moralization of the child as problematical. According to *Freud*, young children are dominated by the id; i. e., they are driven by sexual and aggressive impulses that seek immediate gratification. Infants are unflatteringly described as 'polymorphous perverse', as inherently and relentlessly aggressive and incestuous. Obviously, then, the child's inborn anarchic tendencies must be transformed before he can take his place in society. *Freud*'s creative insight (i. e., that moralization is problematical) was followed by a creative solution. Children's instinctually based incestuous desires, which are directed toward their opposite-sexed parent, inevitably bring them into conflicts with their same-sexed parent. In order to avoid jealous retaliation by a stronger adult, and to avoid displeasing the parent whom he also loves, the child renounces his sexual claims on his opposite-sexed parent and 'internalizes' the image of both mother and father. These internalized images serve thereafter as guides to conduct. Moreover, because the demands of both the instincts and society are relentless, the individual is doomed to a life of internal conflict – too much animal makes a sick society; too much society makes a sick animal.

This much of the conventional psychoanalytic description of moral development is well known. That which is often not recognized are the ambiguous implications of this account, ambiguities that *Freud* himself acknowledged. First, it follows from the Freudian model that he who has internalized the most prohibiting parental model (i. e., he who becomes the most rule-bound) is the most moral. But moral development is clearly not a linear function of the number of rules that a person has incorporated. Rather, from a dialectical viewpoint, being governed by too many or too few rules is equally undesirable. Second, according to *Freud* (1961), the development of conscience is a neurotic defense against the fear of being punished and abandoned by one's parents. Because superego ('moral') anxiety is phenomenally equivalent to neurotic anxiety, moral conduct is essentially a neurotic symptom pattern, a sick compromise we all must make in order to enjoy the benefits of civilized life. Neurotics suffer from an excess of morality, and psychoanalysis, as a consequence, must take an antimoral posture. Once again, however, *Freud*'s analysis seems intuitively unsound. There is a drivenness to neurotic behavior, an absence of the dialectical tension that characterizes authentic moral conduct.

The Role-Theoretical Model

According to *Mead* (1934), a young child is initially egocentric, unable to envision a conflict between his own desires and the needs and goals of others.

However, children are, ultimately, sociable and the dual processes of peer interaction and normal intellectual growth provide them with an increasing ability to comprehend alternative perspectives, including, in particular, the attitudes of others toward themselves. The first signs of this evolution appear when, while a child is engaged in solitary play, he begins to interact with imaginary companions and to adopt the 'viewpoints' of the various toys used in his games. This practice of speaking first in one voice and then another, and of adopting alternating characters in his play, promotes the development of role-taking ability or *empathy*, as it is more simply called. Gradually with the accumulation of role-taking experience, a child becomes able to generalize beyond the context of his immediate social situation. He formulates the viewpoint of the 'generalized other', the expectations that society in the round holds concerning his behavior. According to *Mead*, however, dialectical tension is preserved through a refractory element of individuality known as the 'I', which remains in perpetual opposition to the set of socialized 'me's' that are governed by social expectation. In spite of the polarity that exists between the 'I' and the socialized 'me's', empathy or role-taking ability is for *Mead* the critical aspect of moral development. In fact, *Mead* can be fairly characterized as equating moral development with the emergence of role-taking ability. Although an empathic disposition is clearly necessary for moral conduct, a highly empathic person may, all other things constant, be a moral jellyfish as well as one who is genuinely concerned with the welfare of society. Thus, too much as well as too little empathy can lead to less than moral conduct, and this failure of dialectical perspective is the major flaw in *Mead*'s analysis of moral development.

The Piagetian Model

Piaget (1965) describes moral development as a two-stage process. In the first, the child develops a 'morality of constraint' produced by his experience with unilateral adult authority. In this stage the child accepts parental dictates as moral absolutes – eternal sanctions simply 'given' in nature. The morality of an act is judged in terms of its consequences rather than in terms of the actor's intentions, and justice is equated with whatever the authority commands. Over time the morality of constraint is replaced by a 'morality of cooperation' in which moral rules are seen, not as eternal verities, but as rational conventions which promote orderly social relations. The child becomes independent (i. e., autonomous) of adult sanctions and begins to conceive moral conduct as necessary for the functioning of any social group. The morality of an act is judged in terms of the actor's intentions, and justice is seen in terms of equality and equity. Movement from a heteronomous morality of constraint to an autonomous morality of cooperation is produced by cognitive growth and peer group interaction – the sharing of perspectives with equals.

There are many problems with *Piaget*'s analysis of moral development, two of which will be mentioned. First, as the sociologist *Rieff* (1959) argues, *Piaget*'s discussion of moral development is an attempt to legitimize and reify the old liberal myth that society naturally evolved from a primitive collectivist tyranny to a modern individualist democracy. Second, and more importantly, although *Piaget* defines the morality of cooperation as a multifaceted clinical syndrome, its defining feature is autonomous compliance with social norms. But autonomy is a two-edged concept. That is, if we think in terms of individual differences, one who is at the low end of the autonomy dimension will be pusillanimous and conforming, but one who is at the high end may be either autonomous or autocratic because there is only a fine line between the two.

A Multidimensional Model

In contrast to the moral theories reviewed to this point, the writer takes the position that moral development can be usefully conceptualized in terms of five relatively independent dimensions, and an adequate description of the character structure of any given individual requires taking all five into account (*Hogan*, 1973). The first concerns learning the rules of the social game; this knowledge then provides the rudiments of self-control. The second, socialization, reflects the degree to which a person considers the rules and values of his culture to be personally obligatory and binding. The third dimension is empathy, which provides the capacity to think in terms of the spirit rather than the letter of the law, to consider the implications of one's actions for the welfare of others. The fourth variable is autonomy, the degree to which one's moral decisions are free from the influence of peer group pressures and prestige factors.

The final dimension concerns the degree to which a person considers rules and established procedures as having an instrumental value. One end of this dimension is defined by those who prefer to make decisions on the basis of personal and intuitive moral feelings; these judgments, which are based on the dictates of conscience, may often conflict with established procedures. The opposite pole of this dimension is defined by persons who distrust moral intuitions and prefer instead to rely on conventions, contracts, and formal agreements as a means for regulating social affairs. Considerable evidence is now available which suggests that persons who are at either end of this dimension are less than morally mature. Extreme intuitionists have insufficient regard for the rights and privileges of others. Extreme advocates of the instrumental value of law tend doggedly to defend the *status quo*. And the two positions reflect one of the great dialectical antinomies in the history of legal and social philosophy.

In what sense is this multidimensional model dialectical and developmental? First, according to the model, the ideal endpoint of moral development is moral maturity defined in terms of optimal placement of the five dimensions; the practical endpoint of moral development is social conformance, explained in terms of these dimensions. Furthermore, the appearance of socialization, empathy, and autonomy represents transition points in a person's development which are followed by qualitative changes in the dynamics of social behavior. That is, until a child becomes socialized, he will be egocentric, impulsive, and undisciplined. After socialization but before empathy develops, he will be excessively respectful of adult authority. An empathic but nonautonomous person will place a greater priority on human needs than on the maintenance of rules; however, his conduct will remain closely tied to the expectations of his peer group. It is only after a degree of autonomy has been achieved that behavior may become independent of external controls. In contrast with these three dimensions, moral knowledge and the ethics of conscience – ethics of responsibility continuum are not developmental in the sense described above.

The adjustments to the social environment that a child must make during development are relatively obvious. The major problem for an infant is to secure nurturance and protection. Moreover, as a child becomes mobile, he tends to wander further from his caretaker's protection, thereby exposing himself increasingly to danger. Thus, obedience to commands both facilitates parent-child interaction and improves the child's chances for survival. The primary developmental task for a child in the middle years is to become a social being, a process brought about almost exclusively through peer interaction. For a typical child, such interaction begins around age 4 or 5, where, because adaptation to the group requires accommodation to a radically expanded set of norms, continued strict obedience to parental commands will be maladaptive.

The development of empathy greatly improves the capacity to anticipate and the willingness to comply with the expectations of the group – the prerequisites for sociability – and increases flexibility in peer interaction. Finally, the most important problem for the young adult is to establish his own life-style. Yet most people are caught between the internalized demands of their familiy and the external expectations of the peer community. Thus, the development of autonomy is an important solution to the functional dialectic of development; it allows one to deviate from both parents and peers, but in a (hopefully) prosocial fashion. Seen in this way, the emergence of socialization, empathy, and autonomy is an important solution to the functional dialectic of development; it maturation; they are capacities which mediate both the needs of the individual and the demands of his social group.

Acknowledgment

The author would like to thank S. Karger AG for permission to reproduce this paper. A longer version appeared under its present title in *Human Development 17:* 107–117 (1974). Thanks are also extended to *Esther Blank Greif*, *William Kurtines*, and *Roger Webb* for their helpful comments on an earlier version of this paper.

References

Bandura, A.: Principles of behavior modification (Holt, New York 1969).
Freud, S.: Civilization and its discontents (Norton, New York 1961).
Hogan, R.: Moral conduct and moral character: a psychological perspective. Psychol. Bull. *79:* 217–232 (1973).
Mead, G. H.: Mind, self, and society (University of Chicago Press, Chicago 1934).
Pepper, S. C.: World hypotheses (University of California Press, Berkeley 1942).
Piaget, J.: The moral judgment of the child (Free Press, Glencoe 1965).
Rieff, P.: Freud: the mind of the moralist (Anchor, New York 1959).

Contr. hum. Dev., vol. 2, pp. 60–71 (Karger, Basel 1976)

Chapter 7
Dialectical Operations of Cognitive Development

Klaus F. Riegel[1]

In considering *Piaget*'s (1962, 1963, 1965, 1972) and *Piaget* and *Inhelder*'s (1967) theory and observations of cognitive development, we must surely recognize its dialectic basis. This dialecticism is most clearly revealed in the accommodation-assimilation paradigm leading to adaptation and re-adaptation. Accommodation denotes the changes of the subject to the object, for example, of the observing or eating child. Assimilation denotes the changes of the object to the subject, for example, the shifting into focus of the object visually searched or the physical and chemical changes of the eaten food. In the dialectic sense, both accommodation and assimilation are complementary; they are standing in contradictory relation.

While *Piaget*'s theory is based upon such a dialectic foundation, critics have often wondered how the accommodation-assimilation paradigm is carried forward into the interpretations of the higher stages of cognitive development. Undoubtedly, *Piaget* uses this paradigm skillfully and convincingly for depicting basic biological interactions and early cognitive differentiations, such as sucking, grasping, touching, as well as the coordination and sequencing of these early schemata. Here, *Piaget*'s descriptions resemble the syncretic operations described by *Werner* (1926). As soon as the child reaches the second major period in *Piaget*'s theory, the period of preoperational intelligence, and as soon as *Piaget* shifts from a methodology of observational interpretations to those of experi-

[1] A longer version of this chapter's content appeared under the title 'Dialectic operations: the final period of cognitive development' in *Human Development 16:* 346–370 (1973). The reader is referred to this article for a more detailed consideration of the philosophical, historical, and sociocultural issues involved. The original manuscript was completed during the author's appointment as a Visiting Scholar at the Educational Testing Service, Princeton, N. J. The author is grateful for many constructive comments by *Nancy Datan*, *Walter Emmerich*, *Jack Meacham*, *Ruth Riegel*, *Lee Van den Daele*, and *Bill Ward*. Thanks are extended to S. Karger AG for permission to reproduce this paper.

mentation, the dialectic paradigm of accommodation and assimilation is being neglected and interpretations are proposed in terms of traditional (i. e., demonstrative) logic (see Chapter 1).

For our discussion of the major periods in *Piaget*'s theory, we rely on a much simplified interpretation of cognitive development by *McLaughlin* (1963). At the *sensory-motor* period the child apprehends object permanency, but is not yet able to classify within a dimension; he is able to attend only upon distinct singular objects that happen to come into his field of attention. Neither does he discriminate any of these objects against others nor against negative instances of the same object. For example, the child is able to focus upon a block, but he does not discriminate this block from beads and marbles or non-blocks in general. All that he is able to do is to achieve a figure-ground differentiation. The dialectical character of the early form of cognitive operations is expressed by the fluidity with which the attention of the child might switch from item to item or from figure to ground and from ground to figure.

The dialectical character is also revealed at the next higher level of cognitive operations corresponding to *Piaget*'s period of *preoperational* thought. At this level the child attends to two concepts simultaneously. Thus, he is able to sort items by color into those that are red and those that are green or, more generally, into those which show the presence of an attribute, such as the color red, and those which show its absence, i. e., nonred. The positive and negative instances of an attribute are mutually dependent. Red determines as much that which is not red, as not-red determines red. Both together define the attribute or dimension of discrimination, i. e., color. Such a dimension, at different situations or at higher levels of development, might be contrasted with new alternatives, such as form or materiality.

The discussion of the remaining two developmental periods, the *concrete* and the *formal* operational periods, can be relatively brief. In *McLaughlin*'s simplified interpretation, the child becomes able to operate simultaneously with two attributional dimensions and four concepts, or with three attributional dimensions and eight concepts. Both steps imply important expansions of the child's conceptualization. At the period of concrete intellectual operations, for example, the child succeeds in double classifications and thus can form the logical products A and B, A but not B, B but not A, neither A nor B. At the period of formal operational thought, still further-reaching expansions occur.

All of these operations could be interpreted in a dialectical form if the mutual determination of a class and its inverse, i. e., of the classes A and non-A, were consistently emphasized. While this seems to be obvious enough from a theoretical perspective, in the reports of his research observations, *Piaget* searches systematically for contradictions in the child's judgments, and thereby undermines his own dialectic interpretations as well as he degrades the dialecticity of the child. Of course, *Piaget* merely reports these contradictions and, thus, the dialectically minded reader could use this information adequately to substantiate his own interpretations, but since *Piaget*'s theory subsequently progresses to higher and higher levels at which earlier contradictions are formally resolved, his theory becomes antidialectical and the progress of the child as described by *Piaget* is one of increasing alienation of thought.

Piaget's Theory of Cognitive Development as a Theory of Alienation

Various research reports (see, for example, *Piaget*, 1962, 1963, 1965; *Piaget and Inhelder*, 1967) provide rich sources for demonstrating the dialectical character of the child's thought. The following example shows shifts in the identity concept of a child at an age of 2 years, 7 months: 'J. seeing L. in a new bathing suit, with a cap, J. asked: *What's the baby's name?* Her mother explained that it was a bathing costume, but J. pointed to L. herself and said: *But, what's the name of that?* (indicating L.'s face) and repeated the question several times. But as soon as L. had her dress on again, J. exclaimed very seriously: *It's Lucienne again*, as if her sister had changed her identity in changing her clothes' (*Piaget*, 1962, p. 224).

At an early age, the child is not embarrassed by his own contradictory judgments as shown in the following example on a numerical comparison of sets of items at an age of 6 years and 9 months: 'Are there more wooden beads or more brown ones? *More brown ones*. If we make a necklace with the wooden beads and a necklace with the brown ones, which would be longer? *The one with the wooden beads* (without hesitating). Why? *Because there are the two extra white ones'* (*Piaget*, 1965, p. 176).

Regardless of whether one attributes these contradictory judgments to a change in the child's opinion, to a lack of short-term retention, or to a disability to operate simultaneously with two attributional dimensions, development is seen by *Piaget* (as well as by almost all developmental psychologists) as removing these inconsistencies and as reaching toward a coherent, noncontradictory mode of thinking. These examples also show, however, that thinking originates from a dialectical basis and, as we will try to demonstrate, creative and mature thinking returns to its dialectic mode or rather fails to separate itself from this foundation.

Additional support for our interpretation comes from a study by *Miller* (1972) with the specific purpose of examining children's reactions to the violation of their own expectancies concerning the conservation of weight. Eight- and 10-year-old nonconservers and conservers were studied under conditions where the outcome of the weighing of two clay balls could be overridden by the experimenter, thus creating results inconsistent with the experience of at least the conserving children. Contrary to the investigator's expectation, observable surprise was infrequent and changes in judgment were readily made. Contrary to some earlier findings, active resistance to change was apparent in about half the conservers, but older conservers did not show resistance more often than young conservers.

Miller derives the interpretation of his findings from *Piaget*'s notion of the 'logical necessity' for the persistence of cognitive structures. This notion, in turn, derives from the concept of disequilibration. If a conflict is created through new experiences or cognitive changes, the organism tends to resolve such an incongruity. If such an equilibration is not successfully achieved, the child, especially the younger one, might simply state his observation without persistent attempts to consolidate it with his earlier conceptualization. In *Piaget*'s theory, such a solution represents a regression toward an earlier level of operation. To us, it indicates that the thoughts of the child are flexible enough to tolerate and to exist with ambiguities. Eventually, through alienating training and abstractions, the child will be induced to consolidate these contradictions for the sake of educationally accepted interpretations. In principle, however, these contradictions remain to coexist even within the superimposed structures of later interpretations. Thinking, in the dialectical sense, is therefore the process of transforming contradictory experience into momentary stable structures. These structures consolidate the contradictory evidence but do not represent thinking; they merely represent objectified products of thinking.

Development of Linguistic Operations with Relations

Several studies have explored the acquisition and use of comparative terms, such as 'more' and 'less' or 'tall', 'taller' and 'tallest'. These investigations have been conducted and summarized either by emphasizing a linguistic (*Clark*, 1970) or a perceptual-cognitive basis (*Huttenlocher and Higgins*, 1971). Undoubtedly, the study of comparative terms is intimately related to *Piaget*'s work. In particular, his interpretations of conservation have been criticized for failing to take account of the child's ability to operate and comprehend such terms as 'more', 'less', 'same', etc. (*Griffiths et al.*, 1967; *Donaldson and Balfour*, 1968; *Bickford and Looft*, 1973).

According to the available evidence, simplified to a considerable extent, the following stages in the development of comparative terms may be distinguished. At level 1, when the child is producing single words only, expressions such as 'more' are sometimes used by the child as imperative demands without comparative implications. Paraphrasing his expression, the child seems to say 'I want this here!' At level 2, when the child operates simultaneously with two terms, he might use such words as 'more' in an absolute, dichotomizing manner, contrasting it with 'not more' but not implying a gradient of magnitudes. At level 3, when the child operates simultaneously with three terms, true transitivity and, subsequently, comparativity are established. For instance, the child might apply terms like 'small, medium, tall' or 'tall, taller, tallest'. By dropping off either one of the extreme items of such a series, e. g. A<B<C, he is able to extend it without limitation.

Level 3 represents an important step in an additional sense. All of the previous comparisons implied absolute anchor points. In one-term expressions the condition and desire of the speaker himself serves as an absolute point of reference. In two-term comparisons the expression 'more' serves as the positive instance; 'not more' represents merely its negation. At level 3 the anchor point becomes variable. Applying a spatial representation, usually the left-hand term, as in 'tall, taller, tallest', serves such a function. But by adding new elements at the right, items which were originally the 'tallest' might, finally, appear as relatively short. The same holds for extensions into the left direction, i. e., 'tall', 'less tall', 'least tall'.

At level 4, when the child operates simultaneously with four terms, he ought to be able to make comparisons between two dichotomized variables and perform class multiplications such as between 'wide and narrow versus short and tall'. This performance is one of the logical prerequisites for conservation tasks. Similar performances, although they do not represent any new form of operation, consist of hierarchical comparisons. For example, the child might, first, classify objects into large and small items and, then, subdivide each class in the same manner. This operation, when executed repeatedly, may result in a series in which all items are ordered transitively. Finally, we might expect level 5 and level 6 children to compare simultaneously items along three or more dimensions.

If an object is fast, when compared within a fixed system of coordinates, but slow, when compared with another moving object, we recognize, once more, the dialectical principle of contradiction. This principle implies that a thing has a given quality and, at the same time, does not have it. In regard to comparatives, the statement that something is tall and at the same time small, namely when viewed within two different frames of reference, is equally characteristic of mature judgments. Such a statement cannot be captured easily within a logic of classes and relations.

Proponents of formal logicism might, of course, still claim that these ambiguities could be eliminated if we moved toward systematic quantifications. Instead of saying, for example, that John is taller than Jim, we might state that John is 151 cm and Jim 143 cm tall. This procedure represents, however, a mere regression toward an absolute, arbitrary standard, namely, the Standard Meter in Paris. Moreover, it shows most dramatically, how empty and evasive our thoughts would become if we were to express all our knowledge and opinions in the form of such quantified expressions. As argued elsewhere against modern trends in linguistics (*Riegel,* 1975), the actions of the individual and of society are bound to be based on another foundation, i. e. on a dialectical foundation, and are determined by a concern for the human being rather than by a retreat into formal systematizations.

Dialectical thinking emphasizes the interdependence of form and content. In its narrow sense, it deals with the interrelationship between methods and results, in its most general sense, between subject and object. As one person pronounces a judgment, he externalizes a standard which will direct and modify another person's judgment, which, once it too has been pronounced, will produce further modifications. Thus, these interactions set a process in motion which is in continuous flux and only temporarily at rest, namely, at those moments in which a pronouncement takes place. Such a process of evaluation and reevaluation characterizes the thoughts and judgments of mature persons.

In regard to aged persons it has been proposed that processes of simplification and rigidification have altered their mode of conceptualization and action. But such an evaluation holds only if their thinking is considered to be preceded by all four periods of *Piaget*'s theory and compared against the standards set for the last of these periods, i. e., of formal operations. If dialectical thinking emerges directly from any of the earlier levels of operations, more successful cognitive aging will result. Uncritical adherence to traditional educational and academic goals has made us firmly believe, however, that development has always to proceed through all of the four periods; the further a person advances in his progression, the more successful his development is considered to be. The option to be proposed, which allows that dialectical or mature thinking might emerge from *any* one of the succeeding periods, opens new perspectives for the study and understanding of adult thinking and successful aging (*Riegel*, 1972a, c, 1973).

Cognitive Changes during Adulthood and Aging

Thus far, only two studies of normal-aged subjects have been conducted with tasks taken from the rich repertoire of Piagetian investigations. A few have been made with senile older subjects by *De Ajuriaguerra* (see *Hooper*, 1972); others appeared after this report had been prepared (see especially *Papalia*, 1972).

The two studies reported (*Sanders et al.*, 1966; *Kominski and Coppinger*, 1968) investigated the conservation of surface areas by means of two green cardboards, described as meadows, on which two cows could graze. By placing different numbers of blocks in various positions upon either one or both cardboards, subjects were asked whether equal amounts of grass were available under these different conditions. According to the evidence obtained, older adults do not conserve area as we would expect them and as older children do. They rather seem to have regressed to judgments based on their immediate perceptual impressions, much like those exhibited by younger children.

These results raise the puzzling question of the disappearance of personal knowledge. Let us consider the knowledge of the conservation of matter. Is it conceivable that a person, once he has realized that an amount of liquid remains the same when poured from one beaker into another one of different shape, can ever lose this insight? Do we not always keep knowing what we know?

In one of the two theoretical discussions on cognitive changes during adulthood and aging, *Flavell* (1970) argues for the 'disappearance of knowledge' under conditions of neurophysiological damage. According to available information, such changes are not necessarily affecting all aging persons to a sufficiently severe extent. Arguments against the 'disappearance of knowledge' are based upon the distinction between competence and performance. This distinction has been introduced into linguistics by *Chomsky* and has been translated into cognitive developmental psychology by *Flavell* and *Wohlwill* (1969), though with an emphasis congruent with the traditional distinction in psychology of theoretical constructs and observable behavior.

A second theoretical discussion, focusing upon the transition in cognitive operations from adolescence to adulthood, has been published by *Piaget* (1972). Here *Piaget* seems to weaken his earlier interpretations by giving more attention to individual and societal differences in speed of development, developmental diversification, and professional specialization. Orginally, the four major periods in the cognitive development of the child were regarded by *Piaget* as universal progressions through which all children would move at about the same pace. Studies of cross-cultural and subcultural variations have often failed to confirm such an interpretation and led *Piaget* to suggest that the *speed of progression* is not the same under all social conditions, but may produce retardation in deprived and accelerations in stimulating surroundings. Differences between groups are especially marked at the later periods of development; during the early periods, the progression seems to be most uniform.

Piaget's concessions in regard to individual and social differences are most appropriate. It has never been shown convincingly that the highest level of operation, i. e. formal operational intelligence, characterizes the thinking of mature adults. Only under the most exceptional conditions of logical argumentations and scholastic disputes is it conceivable that a person would engage in such forms of thinking. In his daily activities, logics and operations of much lower power will be applied. Indeed, even in their scientific activities, researchers will very rarely engage in the propositional logic of the fourth period in *Piaget*'s theory and, for example, systematically calculate all possible outcomes in their search for a solution. Creative scientific activities are dominated by playful manipulations of contradictions and by conceiving issues integratively which have been torn apart by formal operational thinking.

For all these reasons, *Piaget*'s theory describes thought in its alienation from its creative, dialectical basis. It represents a prototype reflecting the goals of our higher educational system which, in turn, are reflecting the nonartistic and noncreative aspects in the intellectual history of western man (*Riegel*, 1972b, c). Although, *Piaget*'s theory is founded on a dialectical basis, it fails to make the transition from the formal intellectualism of *Kant* to the concrete dialecticism of *Hegel*. Thus, his theory is not only incapable of interpreting mature thinking but, in his interpretation, also the cognitions of children (increasing with age) lose their dialectical and, thus, their creative character. A commitment to *Hegel* enables us to reinterpret *Piaget*'s theory with due consideration of mature and creative thinking. It leads us to an extension and modification of *Piaget*'s model of cognitive progression.

A Modified Model of Cognitive Development

In a previous publication (*Riegel*, 1972d), we discussed three models of qualitative, developmental changes. These models were derived from the earlier work by *Van den Daele* (1969). In both publications, *Piaget*'s theory of cognitive development was considered to represent the simplest of all three models, the single sequence model. In this model qualitatively different sets of operations or behavior succeed each other in temporal sequence; no provisions for difference in progression between persons or between skills were made nor any statements on the transition and accumulation of behavior across stages. Undoubtedly, this representation oversimplifies the richness of *Piaget*'s theory but, at the present time, there are insufficient reasons for assigning any of the other models, the multiple sequence or the complex sequence model, to represent *Piaget*'s theory.

In view of such an assignment the question arises as to what happens, at later stages, to the behavior or operations acquired and representative of the earlier stages? Are the schemata of the sensorimotor period lost or are they modified and transformed into those of the preoperational and of the higher periods? Moreover, is it conceivable that an individual operates simultaneously at different levels of cognition; perhaps, switching back and forth between them or choosing one for one area of activity and another for another area?

Furth (1973) has maintained that *Piaget* does not 'pretend' that stages of thinking reached in one domain will necessarily be found in the thinking of the same person in another domain' (p. 8). But *Piaget* does not show explicitly that at each stage earlier performances are also executed. As in intelligence testing, he looks only at maximum performances. More importantly, he does not state explicitly the conditions under which switching across stages might occur.

Even if we consider the simplified interpretation by *McLaughlin* (1963), we fail to derive any definite conclusion. The progression depicted in this model represents, as we have seen, a successive increase in the number of attributional dimensions and, thus, in the number of concepts with which a child operates simultaneously. But if a child at the level of preoperational thinking categorizes items according to the presence or absence of one attribute, is he, then, also able to dismiss the attributional dimension altogether and to conceive items 'as such' without any categorizing efforts, i. e., in the manner of the sensorimotor child?

Presumably, the further the child has advanced in his development, the harder it will be to 'regress' to the 'naive' mode of early conceptualization. For this reason, the growth of cognitive organization, as depicted in any of these models, represents an alienation from original thought. Dialectical operations represent a further step forward and, at the same time, a return to early thinking which, in the opinion of many writers (e. g. *Werner, Freud, Zeininger, Levi-Strauss et al.*), is dialectical in nature. All four periods in *Piaget*'s theory represent logical operations and, thus, noncontradictions. This is most obvious at the period of formal operational intelligence. Dialectical operations deny these logical operations at each level; at the formal operational level, the system as such and in its totality is being denied.

As shown in figure 1, we propose that an individual at any developmental level may directly progress to its corresponding mode of dialectical operations,

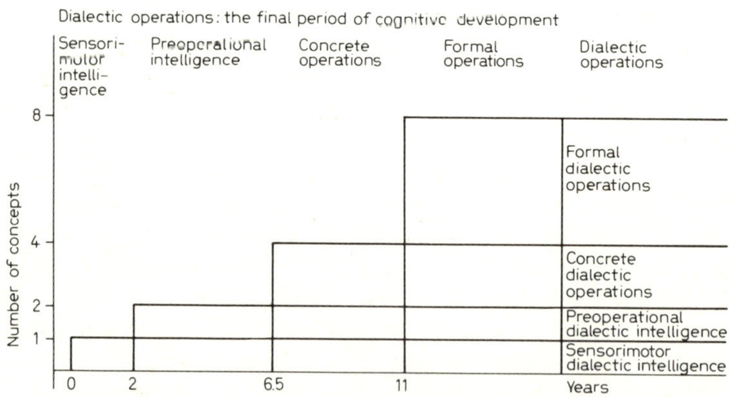

Fig. 1. Schematic representation of five developmental periods for *Piaget*'s extended theory of cognitive development.

reaching thereby a mature stage of thinking. This provision introduces inter-individual variation at the level of maturity. Persons might reach dialectical maturity without ever having passed through the period of formal operations or even through that of concrete operations. This provision also introduces intra-individual variation. The skills and competence in one area of concern, for instance in science, might be of the type of formal dialectical operations; those in a second area, for instance in everyday business transactions, might be of the type of concrete dialectical operations; those in a third area, for instance in artistic activities, might be of the type of preoperational dialectical intelligence; finally, those of intimate personal interactions might be of the sensorimotor and, therefore, of the original dialectical type.

In his discussion of equilibration and disequilibration, *Piaget* touches most explicitly upon the issue of optional, multilevel operations. At the same time, his discussion reveals clearly that his conception of development is one of consecutive alienation. According to *Piaget* as well as to *Lewin* (1954), organisms inherently tend toward equilibrated states. Disequilibrium represents conflict and contradiction which the organism tries to overcome through its activities. The disturbance of the equilibrium is especially marked prior to the transitions from one into the next higher level of operation.

If *Piaget* admits – as *Furth* has declared – that an organism might have implicit or explicit options to operate at different stages of thinking, dependent upon the area of activity with which it happens to be concerned at a particular time, the reliance on the principle of equilibration is weakened if not abandoned. Any concurrent or closely successive operations at different developmental levels ought to create by themselves a state of conflict which ought to be equilibrated. Such an equilibration can only mean the progression to the higher and later developmental level of operation. In other words, the option for multilevel operations contradicts *Piaget*'s notion of equilibration since it reintroduces dialectical conflict; the emphasis upon equilibration would tend to resolve this conflict at the expense of the thinking at the earlier stage. Our own modification recognizes dialectical conflicts and contradictions as a fundamental property of thought. In contrast to *Piaget*, we maintain that at the levels of dialectical operations at maturity, the individual does not necessarily equilibrate these conflicts, but is ready to live with these contradictions; stronger yet, the individual accepts these contradictions as a basic property of thought and creativity.

Conclusion

The purpose of our analysis was to reintroduce dialecticism into *Piaget*'s theory of cognitive development.

We have followed *Hegel*'s (1969a,b) philosophy, especially his *Phenomenology of mind,* which provides an exceptionally rich source and a distinct model of the development of the individual and society. It starts with the delineation of three, essentially cognitive stages but continues with the description of stages of social interactions. Most notably, cognition and social processes are not as firmly separated in *Hegel*'s theory as modern psychologists have come to make us believe.

To this author's knowledge, *Hegel*'s theory has never been seriously explored for psychological interpretations. More convincingly than the dialectical materialists, he has preserved the conception of the active organism by proposing a developmental model in which activities (labor) and products (material) remain in dialectical interdependence. It seems a regression, indeed, if we were to abandon this delicate notion in order to obtain a material underpinning, the significance of which has been recognized in a theory of commodities, products, and economy, but not in a theory of a developing organism within a changing world.

References

Bickford, B. and Looft, W. R.: More on more: the mythology and actuality of children's understanding of relational terms. J. genet. Psychol. *123:* 139–143 (1973).

Clark, H. H.: Comprehending comparatives; in *Flores D'Arcais and Levelt* Advances in psycholinguistics, pp. 294–306 (North-Holland, Amsterdam 1970).

Donaldson, M. and Balfour, G.: Less is more: a study of language comprehension in children. Br. J. Psychol. *59:* 461–471 (1968).

Flavell, J. H.: Cognitive changes in adulthood; in *Goulet and Baltes* Life-span developmental psychology: Research and theory, pp. 247–253 (Academic Press, New York 1970).

Flavell, J. H. and Wohlwill, J. F.: Formal and functional aspects of cognitive development; in *Elkind and Flavell* Studies in cognitive development, pp. 67–120 (Oxford University Press, New York 1969).

Furth, H. G.: Piaget, IQ, and the nature-nurture controversy. Hum. Dev. *16:* 61–73 (1973).

Griffiths, J. A.; Shantz, C. A. and Sigel, I. E.: A methodological problem in conservation studies: the use of relational terms. Child Dev. *38:* 841–848 (1967).

Hegel, G. W. F.: Phänomenologie des Geistes (Suhrkamp, Frankfurt 1969a); The phenomenology of mind (Harper-Torch Books, New York 1967).

Hegel, G. W. F.: Wissenschaft der Logik (Suhrkamp, Frankfurt 1969b); Science of logic (Allen & Unwin, London 1929).

Hooper, F. H.: Cognitive assessment across the lifespan. Methodological implications of the organismic approach; in *Nesselroade and Reese* Life-span developmental psychology. Methodological issues, pp. 299–316 (Academic Press, New York 1972).

Huttenlocher, J. and Higgins, E. T.: Adjectives, comparatives, and syllogism. Psychol. Rev. *78:* 487–504 (1971).

Kominski, C. A. and Coppinger, N. W.: The Müller-Lyer illusion and Piaget's test for the development of the conservation of space in a group of older institutionalized veterans (William and Mary College, Williamsburg 1968).

Lewin, K.: Behavior and development as a function of total situation; in *Carmichael* Manual of child psychology; 4th ed. pp. 918–970 (Wiley, New York 1954).

McLaughlin, G. H.: Psychologic: a possible alternative to Piaget's formulation. Br. J. educa. Psychol. *33:* 61–67 (1963).

Miller, S. A.: Contradiction, surprise, and cognitive change: The effects of disconfirmation of belief on conservers and nonconservers (unpublished, University of Michigan, Ann Arbor 1972).

Papalia, D. E.: The status of several conservation abilities across the life span. Hum. Dev. *15:* 229–243 (1972).

Piaget, J.: Play, dreams, and imitation in childhood (Norton, New York 1962).

Piaget, J.: The origin of intelligence in children (Norton, New York 1963).

Piaget, J.: The child's conception of number (Norton, New York 1965).

Piaget, J.: Intellectual evolution from adolescence to adulthood. Hum. Dev. *15:* 1–12 (1972).

Piaget, J. and Inhelder, B.: The child's conception of space (Norton, New York 1967).

Riegel, K. F.: Development, drop and death. Devl. Psychol. *6:* 306–319 (1972a).

Riegel, K. F.: Developmental psychology and society: some historical and ethical considerations; in *Nesselroade and Reese* Life span developmental psychology: methodological issues, pp. 1–23 (Academic Press, New York 1972b).

Riegel, K. F.: The influence of economic and political ideologies upon the development of psychology. Psychol. Bull. *78:* 129–141 (1972c).

Riegel, K. F.: Time and change in the development of the individual and society; in *Reese* Advances in child development and behavior, vol. 7, pp. 81–113 (Academic Press, New York 1972d).

Riegel, K. F.: On the history of psychological gerontology; in *Eisdorfer and Lawton* The psychology of adult development and aging, pp. 37–68 (American Psychological Association, Washington 1973).

Riegel, K. F.: All the trouble with linguistics. Int. J. Psycholinguist. (in press, 1975).

Sanders, S.; Laurendeau, M., and Bergeron, J.: Aging and the concept of space: the conservation of surface. J. Geront. *21:* 281–285 (1966).

Van den Daele, L. D.: Qualitative models in developmental analysis. Dev. Psychol. *1:* 303–310 (1969).

Werner, H.: Einführung in die Entwicklungspsychologie (Barth, Leipzig 1926). Comparative psychology of mental development (Follett, New York 1948).

Contr. hum. Dev., vol. 2, pp 72–86 (Karger, Basel 1976)

Chapter 8
Chinese Dialectical Thought and Character

Kuo You-yuh[1]

The Chinese uses of dialectical formulations are closely tied to nature, particularly in its developmental aspects. The original author(s) of *I Ching* (also called the *Book of Changes*, Chou dynasty, 1122? –256 BC) proposed that all in nature was the result of two opposing forces: *ch'ien* and *k'un*. *Lao Tzu* (born c. 600 BC) subsequently introduced the terms *yin* and *yang* to account for all of the positive and negative natural phenomena which seemed at play in nature, bringing in thereby a clearly dialectical formulation of events. From this time forward, these two principles of explanation – yin as passive and meek, albeit creative, and yang as active and bold – are used by a succession of different philosophers in the Warring States period (403–221 BC), Ch'in (255–209 BC), and Han (206 BC–220 AD) dynasties to account for the developmental unfolding of historical events.

The style of original Confucian thought, on the other hand, is *not* dialectical. *Confucius* (c. 551–c. 479 BC) was a conservative who attempted to retain and restore the traditional social order of the Chou dynasty. He considered himself a 'transmitter' of social values rather than a creator of them. He laid emphasis on differential (or Confucian) love *(jen)*, propriety *(li)*, and the Rectification of Names *(cheng ming)*. The doctrine of Rectification of Names maintained that once the properties of names – especially titles – were assigned to a person, they acted as standards for his conduct. The individual should therefore play the role implied in the name, as a kind of unipolar designation without variance. This doctrine therefore ignores the growing and changing aspects of the individual or of society, resulting in a constrained and rigid pattern of interpersonal relations. *Chuang Tzu* (c. 370–c. 285 BC), the follower of *Lao Tzu*, chided

[1] *Kuo* is the writer's surname. The writer would like to thank Dr. *Derk Bodde* of the University of Pennsylvania for his critical review of this chapter.

the Confucians for their rigidity and lack of dialectical formulations (*Chuang Tzu,* 1926, chap. 22, pp. 202–283).

Chinese dialecticians are prone to see the harmony in seeming disharmony, as a holistic 'one' among the 'many' inconsistencies, oppositions, negations, etc., of natural existence. Many Chinese philosophers not only thought dialectically about their worlds, but they tried to live in this fashion. They had great tolerance for diversity, which often strikes the Western mind as passive indifference – when it is not! Often they practiced Confucianism in the secular world, while cultivating a more Taoistic or Buddhistic style of life in their spiritual activities.

The latter schools are heavily flavored with dialectical formulations. One finds the philosophical discussions following *Lao Tzu* to center around the possibility of man balancing his secular and spiritual lives. Sometimes the emphasis is put on the spiritual, sometimes on the secular, but in general we find in such philosophies as New-Confucianism a synthesis of Taoism, Buddhism, and Confucianism. This was the predominant philosophical climate before the Communist revolution in China.

Lao Tzu and the Taoistic Way

Though he has never been labeled as such by orthodox Chinese philosophers, *Lao Tzu* must surely be considered China's greatest dialectical philosopher. We might think of him as the Socrates of Chinese thought. Having said this, we must now acknowledge that there are disputes over the actual historical identity of *Lao Tzu*.[2] *Lao Tzu* conceived an ultimate ground in the construction of nature before Heaven and Earth existed (*Tao Te Ching*, 1950, chap. 25, 52).[3] This 'ground' was elusive, evasive (chap. 21), nebulous, silent, invisible, unchanging, unceasing, everrevolving, and standing as One (chap. 25). He did not know its name and called it Tao; if pressed to give a name, he would call it Great (chap. 25). Tao has neither form nor name (chap. 1, 14, 41, 32). It is a Non-

[2] *Fung Yu-lan* (1952, p. 172) believed that the primary author of the *Tao Te Ching* was *Li Erh*, who concealed his doctrines under the name of *Lao Tan*, a legendary figure of the period. However, *Lao Tzu* is generally credited with the authorship of this work, and doubtless his efforts were modified significantly by the editing and rearrangements of subsequent Han scholars. We shall use the collective name *Lao Tzu* to represent the author or authors of the *Tao Te Ching* in the present discussion.

[3] It should be noted that for any one Chinese text there are often several translations available. Some of these go far beyond the original meaning expressed. The writer tried to use as many direct quotations as possible. If a quotation is not direct, chapter sources will be given for easy reference. An effort was made to select the best translation from among many possible sources, so that the reader familiar with this area will find that no one source (e. g., *Lin*'s translation) is used throughout. The various translations employed are listed in the references to this chapter.

Being. 'Non-Being is the origin of Heaven and Earth; and Being is the mother of all things' (*Tao Te Ching*, 1950, chap. 1, p. 1).

Note the view of Non-Being as an active principle. We must not forget that in dialectical logic, an antithesis is just as 'real' as its thesis. In the more demonstrative style of thinking we affirm what 'is' and consider 'what is not' the lack of something (refer to Chapter 1). But this is not true of dialectical reasoning and we see here in *Lao Tzu*'s formulation a fine example of the holistic theory of nature made possible through considering Non-Being as 'something'.

In ancient times agriculture was the major concern. The actions of Earth, where everything is born, were passive and at the mercy of Heaven – as in the case of the rain and sunshine which brought forth sustenance in plant and animal life. Heaven was therefore seen as yang and Earth as yin. In fact, the analogy was drawn between man (yang) and woman (yin), suggesting a form of natural copulation eventuating in the 'impregnation' or fructification of the world. Since there is something invisible which gives birth to everything, *Lao Tzu* could not give it a name, so he called it Tao. It is this having to deal with what-is-not in order to account for what 'is' that *Lao Tzu* speaks of when he observes that 'Everything in the world generates from Being, and Being from Non-Being' (*Tao Te Ching*, 1950, chap. 40, p. 74). In other words, Non-Being has the potential for 'motherhood'.

Tao is also given developmental emphasis through this dialectical communication of the yin and yang principles: 'Tao creates One; One creates Two; Two creates Three; out of Three, All things are created' (*Tao Te Ching*, chap. 42, p. 78). Progression and advance occur dialectically. The allusions here are generally framed in terms of motherhood. Tao is the Mother of all mothers and is 'the mysterious secret of the universe' (*Tao Te Ching*, 1950, chap. 62. p. 114). Out of one comes two, which in turn leads to replacement of the old thing by a new and higher thing. The dynamics of Tao involved here lie in the contradiction innate in things.

The already mentioned 'seeming' passivity of the Chinese character stems from an appreciation of the 'other side' of action or force – we might say, the yin side. It takes a dialectical orientation towards life to appreciate the great *power* contained in the force of passivity. *Lao Tzu* (*Lin*, 1948, chap. 78, p. 143) liked to point out that a very malleable, 'weak' thing like water can wear away the most rock-hard substances in time. Thus, rather than passive out of weakness, the ideal character among the Chinese people would be one which was 'weak-but-actually-strong'. Chinese heroic figures created in some popular novels are portrayed as submissive, probably weak and contrite in appearance, calm, etc., but when provoked to a fight they exhibit the skills of a superman. But even the ideal of combat is to avoid a kind of brutish attack. One utilizes the opponent's hostile thrust against him, or, strikes a kind of 'total' blow – as in the hurricane's pervasive force – which cannot be located but happens so abruptly as to appear 'undelivered'. In this sense, we might say that the Chinese affirm yin principles in their character ideals, yet they would not 'turn the other cheek' indefinitely.

But it is doubtless true that themes of harmony predominate in Chinese writings. *Lao Tzu* (*Lin*, 1948, chap. 2, p. 47) amplified the beauty of harmony by pointing out the interdependence of contraries, as follows:

> Being and Non-Being interdependent in growth;
> Difficult and easy interdependent in completion;
> Long and short interdependent in contrast;
> High and low interdependent in harmony;
> Tones and voice interdependent in harmony;
> Front and behind interdependent in company.

Lao Tzu frequently addressed himself to the question of 'not regarding self as self' (*Lin*, 1948, chap. 7, 13, 19). The Sage must act, but not appropriate, accomplish, but claim no credit (*Lin*, 1948, chap. 2). A person with this kind of loving attitude toward others is more likely to transcend interpersonal antagonism and harmonize (accept, tolerate) diversity in outlooks among men. The sentiment of yielding and losing bears the semblance of a kind of metamotivation, whereby the dynamics of growth are actuated and harmony is established between the opposing forces of contradiction through selfless and unconditional love. This selfless orientation was especially clear in ancient Chinese art (*Hsu*, 1953). Nature is always placed above the individual, who is depicted as miniscule in the scheme of things.

The Ch'anist Way of Dialectical Transcendence

Taoism and Buddhism

Lao Tzu's concept of Non-Being together with *Chuang Tzu*'s Great Sameness (one in many) paved the way for the Chinese to accept Mahāyāna Buddhism from India. In fact, Mahayana Buddhism was greatly enriched by Taoistic concepts and was thereby further branched into several different 'schools' in China. Among these schools, Ch'an Buddhism is considered typically Chinese and was introduced to Japan known as Zen Buddhism. Dialectical themes pervade all these schools of Buddhism.

There are some fundamental differences in world outlook between Taoism and Ch'an Buddhism. The ultimate principle in Taoism is Non-Being, whereas in Ch'an Buddhism it is Void. As we have already noted, Non-Being produces Being; but Void is said to neither increase nor decrease for it is a complete emptiness. Taoism emphasizes Nature (or Spontaneity) whereas Ch'an Buddhism emphasizes Mind (or 'Original Nature'). Taoism, thus, sees man as part of nature, as truly existing within natural events. Ch'an Buddhism, on the other hand, considers all such manifestations to be temporary and illusory. From the mundane point of view, what we as human beings see and feel seems to change and to that extent can be termed 'Being'. But from the more accurate and absolute point of view, sensations are 'Non-Being' because they are illusory.

Thus, in Chinese Buddhism, Being and Non-Being are artificial designations of the two sides of things; these are not truly dialectical aspects of existence. We find the more true dialectical treatment here in such questions as permanence versus change, or of Being-Non-Being versus the denial of both Being and Non-Being. In a sense, Buddhistic philosophy seeks a 'permanence' in existence, without beginning or end – a kind of eternal balance not unlike the classless state of *Marx* or the enlightened monarchy conception of *Hegel*. That is, Buddhists essentially end the dialectical development in the state of Original Nature (or Mind), which means that all contradictories are resolved and tensions cease due to the oneness a Buddhist monk achieves with nature.

Middle Path: A Way of Transcendence

Buddhism originated as an effort to transcend a sort of dialectical 'fate'. *Siddhartha Guatama* (563 BC? –443 BC?), the Indian founder of Buddhism, saw the people of his time suffering from the painful contrasts of life and death, rich and poor, love and hate, war and peace, etc., and decided to frame a way of transcending these harmful bifurcations. His solution was to deny everything in this world and to prepare oneself for the 'other' world (hereafter). This nonharmonious interpretation of dialectical contradiction is also evidenced in Chinese Buddhism. *Chih-k'ai* (538–597 AD), the founder of the *T'ien-t'ai* school of Buddhism, felt that the storehouse of the *Tathāgata* (*Ju-lai*, or *Buddha*) embodies two kinds of nature – i. e., one pure, the other impure (*Fung*, 1952, p. 379). Although both existed within mind, pure nature follows mind but impure nature does not. The result was a kind of internal state of dialectical contradiction. Here was another view of a 'clash' variety calling for some kind of resolution. Gradually, a certain application of dialectical themes in Buddhism permitted a negation of such oppositions to emerge as the 'Middle Path'.

We see this in the views of *Hui-neng* (638–713), the sixth patriarch of Ch'an Buddhism. In the last chapter of the book, *Sūtra Spoken by the Sixth Patriarch*, *Hui-neng* (1929) outlined thirty-six pairs of opposites such as yin and yang, water and fire, good and evil, etc., and advised his disciples to employ dialectical tactics in their teaching. The point here was *not* to resolve the antitheses through synthesis, but rather to *negate* the extremes of dialectical opposition. *Hui-neng* held, as a higher form of 'Absolute Truth', that we must (dialectically) negate the contradictions implied in such dialectical oppositions such as 'good-bad'. In a sense, this is like the Hegelian-Marxian 'negation of a negation'. If we accept good *and* bad as existent, we are bound to these contradictions, literally a slave to their import. But when we deny these extremes, we are free to take the Middle Path (termed Nirvana in Indian Buddhism).

The Orthodox Way

I Ching and Dialectical Development

Thus far we have been considering the writing of the *Tao te Ching,* but as noted in the introduction to this chapter, the *I Ching* was also an influential classical text. Its themes were emphasized by New-Confucianism, which was the official philosophy of all Chinese governments preceding the Communist Revolution – making it the orthodox view. *Chu Hsi* (1130–1200) was its chief architect in the AD period. The *I Ching* was also influential in the New Text School, founded primarily by *Tung Chung-shu* (179? –104 BC). Recall that the *I Ching* had the parallel conceptions to yin and yang in the meanings of ch'ien (yang, masculine) and k'un (yin, feminine). Indeed, the *'I'* of *'I Ching'* is comparable to *Lao Tzu*'s conception of Tao, as a 'Great Ultimate' which produced the two opposing, dialectical principles.

The fascinating aspect of the *I Ching*'s use of dialectic is that it closely parallels the form of dialectical progression we see in the Hegelian and Marxian formulations of 'thesis-antithesis-synthesis', leading in turn to a further round of this sort when the synthesis becomes a new thesis. In the *I Ching* a metaphor of the door was used, as follows:

> A door shut may be pronounced [analogous to] *k'un* [yin, or inactive condition], and the opening of the door *ch'ien* [yang, or active condition]. The opening, succeeding being shut, may be pronounced a change; and the passing from one of those states to the other may be called the constant course [of things] (*I Ching,* The Great Appendix, 1935, sec. I, chap. 11, p. 298).

The yang or ch'ien principle may be seen as the initiating affirmation or 'thesis' in the sequence of developmental events. The yin or k'un principle, on the other hand, was not interpreted in quite as 'contradictory' a fashion as was the antitheses of the Hegelian-Marxian dialectic.

There is an aspect of the *I Ching*, which is not to be seen quite so boldly in the *Tao Te Ching*, and this has to do with the notorious distinction between the male and female status in neo-Confucianism. As we have already said, Confucian philosophy was not dialectical in outlook, but comes much closer to the more demonstrative styles of thought to be seen in the West. However, in neo-Confucian thought a greater emphasis was given to oppositional factors in human relations, if for no other reason than the historic tendency to equate yang and yin with male and female. There was also the natural tendency to bring together themes from *Lao Tzu* and the *Tao Te Ching* with those of the *I Ching*. In any case, thanks to this wedding of dialectical to Confucian thought, a tendency in the *I Ching* exists which elevates the yang principle as more active, hence more noble, honorable, and akin to Heaven. The yin principle is analogized to Earth, as low and mean. This kind of emphasis meshed well with Confucian ideas on the structure of the family, with the male as head of the household and woman as his 'lesser' counterpart. But even within-sex comparisons favored yang. In the fourth chapter of the Great Appendix of *I Ching*, yang (ch'ien) is equated with the way of Superior Men, and yin (k'un) with that of the Small Man.

It is difficult for a Westerner to appreciate the pervasiveness of yin-yang thinking in the Chinese outlook. Not only were natural, social, historical, and individual events interpreted from this perspective, but even Chinese medicine took its origins from the Taoistic yin-yang world view (*Chang*, 1971, pp. 41–44). This approach to medicine classifies the symptoms of disease into dialectically derived categories, such as surface-inside, solidness-void, and so forth. These dimensions were further subsumed under two major dialectical conceptions: coldness and hotness. Coldness refers to the deterioration of basal metabolism; hotness refers to its acceleration. Based on these premises, the 'cold-hot therapy' of China tries to heat the body when cold, cool it when hot, compensate it when it is void, evacuate it when it is solid, and so forth. Although far removed from the usual conception of yin and yang, in point of fact the underlying dialectical formulation here is clear.

Harmonizing the Dialectical Contradiction through Love

Rather than the clash and possible 'explosion' of a Marxian 'class warfare' variety to be seen in Western dialectical formulations, the Chinese have emphasized the harmonic totality of yin and yang. These are not different 'identities' but harmonious aspects of a given 'oneness' *(Tao, I)*. A historian quoted in *Kuo Yü* (*Fung*, 1952, p. 32) drew the distinction between harmony and identity which underwrites much of Chinese thinking on opposition. Harmony is a synthetic function resulting in the production of new things; identity simply adds up the things that have already existed into varying frequencies of 'this' or 'that' variety. The gain to be seen in identity is thus quantitative, so that increasing the number of identities on one side tilts the balance of power and thereby is more likely to generate clash. Harmony, on the other hand, brings about qualitative changes in what currently exists through the synthesizing of differences as a totality. We do not add to one side at the expense of the other in harmony, but rather rearrange what is available for both sides to benefit from.

In a true sense, this harmonizing principle is one of *love*, and it is therefore not surprising that *Fang* (1957, pp. 75–76), an eminent Chinese philosopher, extracted a principle of love from the *I Ching* which may be taken as a force of harmony in the yin-yang relationship:

> What is here called love is just the *intimate communion* [italics added] in intensified emotional contrasts like the conviction of opposite electrical charges across a spark-gap. It is

a universal process wherein Heaven and Earth lead all things to play important parts in the sport of bliss. The strong and the tender supervene upon each other concordantly . . . In a word, life of all forms is fulfilled and value of all kinds is achieved through the spirit of love.

New-Confucianism in the History of China

Before turning to Maoist thinking, we might now survey a few other dialectical theories in the neo-Confucian line of descent. We do so in order to underscore the importance given to this style of thought in China's history before the onset of the Communist Revolution there. *Tung Chung-shu* (179? –104 BC) used the yin-yang principle to interpret both seasonal movements and human affairs. He took the typical neo-Confucian outlook which favored cultivation of yang, which he equated with goodness and the relative de-emphasis of yin, which he equated with covetousness. *Tung* held that in the spring of the year yang forces move from out of the east to oppose yin forces emanating from the west. There is a gradual movement to the south at the time of summer for both forces, but in this case yang gains more power and is ascendant over yin. This supremacy of yang brings about growth in nature, plant life, and so forth. As the yin and yang pass by in the course of the year, yang tends to lose power in its westward flow and yin increases in power as it reaches the east. This is the autumn period. Yin then reaches its peak in the winter months, when the two forces move northward as a kind of mirror-opposite pattern to the southern flow we have outlined in the summer. Yin thus destroys vegetation and halts growth in the frigid season. But, thanks again to the continuing flow in opposition to each other, yin and yang find themselves moving once again into position for spring as the cycle repeats itself in the following year.

In human behavior, the yang and yin forces were said by *Tung* to be active in 'human nature' and 'desire', respectively.[4] Human nature (yang force) manifests itself in the virtues of Confucianistic love *(jen)*, but desire or covetousness *(t'an)* is also true of human behavior (yin force). As with *Tung*'s interpretation of the seasons, the relationship between yin and yang is not always harmonious in the human breast. One force can suppress the other, and since yang was said to be on the side of Heaven and yin on the side of Earth, there was a kind of morality implied in human relations. In order to come closer to Heaven, man must repress the yin force and cultivate the yang force. Indeed, behaving this way literally causes Heaven to increase a 'yang atmosphere' in which man's 'earthiness' (immorality) would necessarily be diminished (i. e., yin would be

4 The word we translate here as 'desire' is *ch'ing,* which also has the meaning of emotion, sentiment, and feeling. In the Chinese language, emotion *(ch'ing)* and desire *(yü)* can be used as a compound word. Since *Tung* considered *ch'ing* to be covetousness, and since he also equated this to desire, we take the liberty of translating this work as desire rather than the more general term 'emotion'.

checked). This idea of repressing one's baser yin-desires in favor of a supposedly higher yang love *(jen)* is referred to as stoicism in Chinese philosophy.

The yin-yang philosophy and stoicism were furthered by *Chou Tung-yi* (1017–1073) of the Sung dynasty. He is noted for his work on *T'ai-chi T'u (Diagram of the Supreme Ultimate)* and the text which explained the movement of yin and yang in terms of hexagrams in the *I Ching*. *Chou* held that the constant alternation, interaction, and unification of yin and yang were said to produce the five *ch'is* (vital forces) of water, fire, wood, metal, and earth. Though he emphasized the yang over the yin principle, *Chou* strongly advised that societal as well as human relations be cultivated in a harmonious fashion. This is possible only through eliminating selfish desire from our natures. *Chou* liked to speak of the 'singleness' which a Sage must achieve if he is to experience perfect harmony. Singleness meant desirelessness, which in turn led to a state of vacuity. Vacuity is like a shining mirror, which reflects all things (a 'one' reflecting the 'many' as a totality of harmony).

Chou Tung-yi was followed by a series of neo-Confucian philosophers, including *Chang Tsai* (1020–1077), *Ch'eng Hao* (1032–1085), *Ch'eng Yi* (1033–1108) and *Chu Hsi* (1130–1200). We have already mentioned *Chu Hsi* above, as the chief architect of neo-Confucianism. Educated in Taoism and Confucianism, *Chu* combined the tenets of both these views in his philosophy. We see the familiar dialectical style of conceptualization in his *li* and *ch'i* constructs. *Li* is an archetype, lying behind and governing all movement and quiescence in the world. *Ch'i* is the manifestation or realization of this archetype in literal movements or actual states of quiescence. These two are one, but it is also true that there would be nothing without some precedent *li* acting as prototype to bring about (via *ch'i*) its actuality. This philosophy is reminiscent of the Socratic-Platonic philosophy, in which a realm of Being was said to house pure ideas or 'ultimates'. *Chou* called this the Supreme Ultimate. If one could but grasp the *li* of the Supreme Ultimate, he would enjoy a sudden enlightenment and come to understand every *li* at play in the world of experience. Also consistent with the Socratic-Platonic philosophy is *Chou*'s observation that 'there is nothing isolated in [experience], and everything must have its opposite' (*Needham*, 1953, p. 466).

The Maoist Way

Our review of the yin-yang doctrine makes it clear that it has changed very little from the time of its inception in the Chou dynasty (1122? –256 BC). This relational way of thinking and speaking about existence, reflected in the Chinese language *per se* (*Kuo*, 1971b, pp. 181–184), was to provide a background of ready acceptance for the Communistic dialectical conceptions of *Mao Tse-tung*.

Mao's thought is highly complex, reflecting decided westernized tendencies yet retaining always that stamp of Eastern Man. His political outlook seems related historically to the Chinese concept of an equalitarian society. His 'methodology' outlook is more directly in line with westernized views. His dialectical orientation is mainly Chinese, but *Mao*'s psychology of knowledge and outlook on human behavior is heavily westernized. We see this in his treatise *On Practice* (*Mao*, 1967a pp. 285–310). Only through practice (learning by doing and by participating in productive and political activities, etc.) can man gain true knowledge, and this takes place in three stages. The first is the perceptual stage of cognition. At this level, man sees only the phenomenal side to things, the separate and disjointed aspects and external relations in events. Through repeated practice at the level of sense perceptions and impressions, a change takes place in the brain, so that – usually occurring suddenly – an added insight becomes possible. This is the second stage, and at this level the person can see the totality of things, including their internal relations. Concepts are formed at this point. Finally, in the third stage, which is called the stage of rational knowledge, man is said to be capable of drawing inferences and making judgments.

This input, constitutive form of theory is very much in line with the thinking of British philosophy, and has been termed a 'Lockean Model' of theoretical description (*Rychlak*, 1973, p. 10). It is due to a model of human behavior of this sort that *Mao*'s social practices stress the importance of people doing (i. e., practicing) that which is considered essential to the mastery of knowledge, and the maintenance of a proletarian spirit. The so-called 'cultural revolution' of the 1960s reflects this philosophy of countering the then emerging bureaucratic class by urging the proletarians to reeducate the new class which threatened to emerge. As an antidote to alienation when proletarians become the ruling class, *Mao* recommended self-criticism and group-criticism as a form of self-negation without the finality of a violent class struggle. But only through constant practice of some such techniques, urging others, looking into ourselves, can we hope to sustain the benefits of the Communistic Revolution.

We find some striking parallels between *Mao*'s *On Contradiction* (1967b) and historical Chinese texts. Not only did he make statements reminiscent of *Hui Shih*'s 'paradox' of the interdependence of subjective and objective meanings (*Chuang Tzu*; 1926, p. 18), but he also quoted the famous Chinese historian of the Han dynastiy, *Pan Ku*, as follows:

> We Chinese often say, 'Things that oppose each other also complement each other.' That is, things opposed to each other have identity . . . 'oppose each other' refers to the mutual exclusion or the struggle of two contradictory aspects. 'Complement each other' means that in given conditions the two contradictory aspects unite and achieve identity. Yet struggle is inherent in identity and without struggle there can be no identity (*Mao*, 1967b, p. 343).

Mao used this commentary to support his view of identity as a form of quasi-Taoistic totality containing within it contradictory aspects that could well reverse positions into their opposites even as the over-all unity was retained. *Mao* viewed motion as taking place in two stages. The first stage of motion is *quantitative*, in which a temporary unity of opposition has been achieved, so that we are likely to misconstrue such states as unity, solidarity, harmony, balance, etc., as lacking in change since they appear 'at rest'. However, when the underlying dialectical oppositions are so rearranged as to dissolve this unity, we have the second stage – of a *qualitative* motion – taking place. The implication of this view is that an underlying struggle between opposite forces can exist in a society, even as the total society seems to be in equilibrium.

The particular struggle which takes place depends upon the nature of the underlying dialectical contradiction. Some contradictions in a society are characterized by open antagonism, others by temporary interdependence. In fact, internal struggles of this type take place within as well as between political parties, and they also are to be seen in the internal psychology of the individual. Extending the Marxian dialectic, *Mao* now sees the single human being as constantly in the process of dialectical change based upon various internal contradictions in his very psychic nature. As already noted above, to resolve contradictions within one's identity, or, within one's political party, *Mao* advocated self-criticism and open exchanges, in what a Westerner might consider a form of 'group encounter'. This is a significant departure from classical Marxian theory, since *Mao* is suggesting that the dialectical process does *not* end via some final 'negation of a negation' into the classless state *for all time!* Dialectical exchanges go on, winnowed down now from the broader class struggle to struggles within a common party outlook, or struggles of conflicting inclinations within a single person.

This idea of contradictions existing in all things is reminiscent of the yin-yang doctrine. *Mao*'s (1967b, pp. 311–347) theory of causation follows the classical view of developmental change via dialectical confrontation. Those 'efficient causes' we see taking place in material events were considered secondary causes by *Mao*. It is the underlying dialectical opposition in all things which provides the actual thrust for change as a 'primary cause'. As *Mao* (1976b, p. 313) expressed it:

> Thus materialistic dialectics effectively combats the theory of external causes, or of an external motive force ... purely external causes can only give rise to mechanical motion, that is, to changes in scale or quantity, but cannot explain why things differ qualitatively in thousands of ways and why one thing changes into another.

Mao was careful to emphasize that his theory did not *exclude* the functioning of external or 'mechanistic' causes. Such causes are important to the motion we termed above 'quantitative'; but *Mao* wished to account for qualitative motion and therefore said that 'external causes are the condition of change and internal causes are the basis of change . . . external causes become operative through internal causes' (*Mao*, 1976b, p. 314). This tendency on his part to stress the continuing interaction between internal and external is very similar to the Chinese tradition in philosophy of emphasizing the relations and interactions between all things.

Mao believed in two kinds of contradictions: universal and particular. He spoke of universal contradictions as follows: 'Contradiction is present in all processes of objectively existing things and of subjective thought and permeates all these processes from beginning to end; this is the universality and absoluteness of contradiction' (*Mao*, 1976b, p. 345). As examples of this kind of contradiction, *Mao* quoted from *Engels'* writing in which things like action and reaction, positive and negative electricity, combination and dissociation of atoms, and the class struggle were cited as universal contradictions. On the other hand, said *Mao*, the contradiction in each form of motion in matter has its particular quality which distinguishes it from other contradictions. The quality of such contradictions can differ from matter to matter, or from interpersonal relation to interpersonal relation. In the final analysis, the ultimate universality of contradiction resides in its *particularity*. The qualitative differences which result from such multiplicity are what give life its color and continuing motive force for change.

A practical outcome of this view of the particularity of contradiction is that human beings are *not* to be lumped into one bland category – which is the view many Westerners have of Chinese society. At least in principle, *Mao* held that the particularity of contradiction must lead in time to educational practices and political decisions which take individual differences into account. As a matter of fact, the psychologists in China have been encouraged to conduct more researches on individual differences (*Kuo*, 1971a, pp. 95–105). The particularity of contradiction thesis also permits us to view each new motion or change in the culture as somehow unique. This is so because one cannot simply apply solutions of yesterday to the changing circumstances of today. There must be a specific method to solve each specific problem in the course of development, rather than some one routine methodology to deal with all contingencies.

A practical example of how *Mao*'s thought on contradiction is utilized in China appeared in the publication *China Pictorial* (1970). A group of scientists in an Auxiliary Food Administration near Peking discovered that three tomatoes had retained their freshness within a batch of spoiled tomatoes. These three tomatoes had been stored for over 1 month. Now, according to *Mao*'s theory, the contradictions contained within the three healthy tomatoes were also contained in the others. Why then did they survive? According to *Mao* (1976b, p. 332):

> . . . if in any process a number of contradictions exist, only one of them is the principal contradiction playing the leading and decisive role while the rest occupy a secondary or

subordinate position. So in studying any process – if it is a complicated process in which more than two contradictions exist – we must do our utmost to discover its principal contradiction. Once the principal contradiction is grasped, any problem can be readily solved.

Based on this reasoning, the scientists began a study of the contradictions among temperature, humidity, and ventilation. They reported that it was the contradiction between temperature and ventilation which determined the rate of spoilage, with temperature acting as the major thrust (the 'thesis' or 'yang', so to speak). By adjusting these two factors, the scientists found that they could preserve tomatoes for 2 months. But *Mao's* distinction between internal and external causes led them to carry their investigations even further. Looking to the internal functioning of the tomato, they discovered that after the fruit had been separated from its plant, it continued to exhale carbon dioxide and inhale oxygen to complete its 'late maturation stage'. This finding led them to control the intensity of the tomato's 'breathing', and hence to retard the rate of metabolism – all of which improved their preservation techniques significantly.

Though the Western scientist might have arrived at these findings through his more demonstrative, Lockean strategy of studying the 'elements' rather than the 'contradictions' in events, the point of this mundane example is to show how dialectical reasoning strategies can be translated into and guide empirical investigations which prove instructive and helpful. Dialectical reasoning is a highly supple, creative form of thinking, and it doubtless enters into the approaches of *all* scientists, who then in turn 'firm up' their insights by a more demonstrative strategy of proof (refer to Chapter 1).

Conclusions and Implications

We have tried in the present chapter to pull together several earlier dialectical Chinese philosophies and to show how they had prepared the way for a form of Communistic theory in present-day China which is only partially identical to the dialectical formulations of Western Communism. In the Hegelian-Marxian dialectics, framed as they were *predominantly* in terms of clash and unresolvable contradictions, it was more likely that a conversion of the dialectic into the Enlightened Prussian Monarchy *(Hegel)* or the classless state *(Marx)* would have to take place. In a sense, the predicate assumptions made by *Hegel* and *Marx* dictated that someday dialectical developments must end. Mao, on the other hand, gave his theory of the dialectic a more indigenous totality, thanks to the antecedent Chinese philosophies of the 'one' among 'many' that constituted all things. He brought the dialectic down to the interpersonal level once the Revolution was completed, keeping it alive and ensuring that it would for all time provide the motive power for advance, self-reflexivity, creativity, individuality, and so forth. This, we feel, is a definite difference between Eastern and Western theories of Communism.

If we now look at what American and other newspaper reporters have said of modern China, and particularly of its people, we find that they use terms like selflessness, stoicism, hardworking, and camaraderie to describe the Chinese character. An American President (Ford) even used the youth of China as an example worthy of emulation in a talk he gave to the graduating class of an American University in 1974. We can find all of these characterological values emphasized in the traditional dialectical philosophies of China. Neo-Confucianism stressed filial loyalty, and in modern times this has been extended to all people – in a neighborhood, for example. The writer contends that it is this traditional enjoyment of brotherhood, and not Communism, which makes the new Chinese character so drawn to the cultivation of camaraderie. The stoicism and selflessness take us back to the Taoism mentioned in the present chapter. The so-called 'submission to the state' which some Westerners see Communism 'bringing about' in China is in actuality a continuation of the historical tendency for man to humble himself before nature – and society is thus seen as an extension of nature's dialectical development. In short, all of the 'newly emerging' characteristics of the Chinese people seen today are not so new. They have been presaged and determined in large extent by the dialectical worldview that has always been intrinsic to the Chinese mentality.

References

Chang, Kung-jang: The pulse-feeling of Chinese medicine. Ming Pao Mon. *6/9:* 41–44 (1971).

China Pictorial: vol. 2/284, pp. 13–14 (1970).

Chuang Tzu: Chuang Tzu: 2nd ed.; transl. by Giles (Kelly & Walsh, Shanghai 1926).

Fang, Thomé H.: The Chinese view of life (The Union Press, Hong Kong 1957).

Fung, Yu-lan: A history of Chinese philosophy, vol. 1; transl. by Bodde (Princeton University Press, Princeton 1952).

Hsu, F. L. K.: Americans and Chinese: two ways of life (Schuman, New York 1953).

Hui-neng: Sūtra spoken by the sixth patriarch on the high seat of 'the treasure of the law' (in Chinese), preface dated 1290 (Buddhist Book Distributor, Hong Kong 1929).

I Ching (in Chinese) in *Sung* The text of Yi King and its appendices: a Chinese original with English translations (The China Modern Education, Shanghai 1935).

Kuo, You-yuh: Psychology in Communist China. Psychol. Rec. *21:* 95–105 (1971a).

Kuo, You-yuh: Family constellation in the Chinese languages. J. indiv. Psychol. *27:* 181–184 (1971b).

Lin Yutang: The wisdom of Lao Tze (Modern Library, New York 1948).

Mao, Tse-tung: On practice (1937); in Selected works of Mao Tse-tung, vol. I, pp. 295–310 (Foreign Languages Press, Peking 1967a).

Mao, Tse-tung: On contradiction (1937); In Selected works of Mao Tse-tung, vol. I, pp. 311–347 (Foreign Languages Press, Peking 1967b).

Needham, J.: Science and civilization in China, vol. I (University Press, Cambridge 1953).

Rychlak, J. F.: Introduction to personality and psychotherapy: a theory-construction approach (Houghton Mifflin, Boston 1973).

Tao Te Ching (in Chinese) Hsuan-Feng, Taipei 1950.

Contr. hum. Dev., vol. 2, pp. 87–100 (Karger, Basel 1976)

Chapter 9
Facts and Dialectics

Steinar Kvale

> Das Höchste wäre: zu begreifen, dass alles Factische schon Theorie ist.
>
> Goethe

> In the 'facts' we find the crystallisation of the essence of capitalist development into an ossified, impenetrable thing alienated from man.
>
> Lukacs

With the frequent appeal to facts in psychology today, one might also expect some reflection upon the nature of facts. However, the question 'what is a psychological fact?' is seldom heard. By analyzing the apparently simple concept of fact in the present chapter, some essential contradictions of psychology as a science can be revealed. The present approach fully acknowledges the positive furthering of a scientific psychology by collecting and analyzing facts of human behavior. Its theme of focus is, however, the question of whether the current scientistic 'cult of the fact' hampers the obtainment of a truly scientific knowledge of behavior. When not otherwise indicated, the concepts of facts and data are used synonymously.

The Manifest Structure of Data

Some assumptions implied in the behavior of observing and collecting psychological data shall be suggested here. A few are explicitly stated in textbooks on scientific methodology, while others remain tacit presuppositions.

Data are *isolated* fragments of a behavioral process.

Data are *unequivocal*. Data do not contain ambiguities or contradictions; they are certain and definite, not to be doubted.

Data are *immutable*, they no longer develop or change.

Data are *intersubjectively reproducible*. Data are those aspects of behavior about which observers can agree.

Data are *externally related* to each other. Data do not involve internal relations between the different aspects of a unity.

Data are *quantifiable*. The multitude of qualitative aspects of behavior reduce to those dimensions which can be measured and calculated, which can be counted as more-or-less.

Data are *given*. Data are immediately experienced, they are not based on the intuitions or speculations of an observer.

Data *appear* directly. Data belong to the surface of a phenomenon, not to its essence.

Data are *abstract*. Data involve an abstracting of isolated elements from their original concrete social and historical situation.

Data are *value-neutral*. Facts are statements of what is factually given, and do not involve value judgments; they are descriptive and not normative.

The Theoretical Context of Facts: Empiricism

The belief that science shall be built on facts and data has been central in empiricist and positivist philosophy. The structure of empiricist thought has succinctly been formulated as follows:

> The metaphysical or vulgar evolutionist world outlook sees things as isolated, static and one-sided. It regards all things in the universe, their forms and their species, as eternally isolated from one another and immutable. Such change as there is can only be an increase or decrease in quantity or a change of place. Moreover, the cause of such an increase or decrease or change of place is not inside things but outside them, that is, the motive force is external ... They contend that a thing can only keep on repeating itself as the same kind of thing and cannot change into anything different ... Consequently, they can explain neither the qualitative diversity of things, nor the phenomenon of one quality changing into another (*Mao Tse-tung*, 1968, p. 25).

In this meaning of metaphysics, there is nothing as metaphysical as an empiricist fact..

The British empiricist philosophy developed by *Hobbes, Locke* and *Mill* conceived of knowledge as founded upon elementary sense-data. Consciousness consisted of isolated sensedata or sensations, as basic atoms which were externally connected by mechanical associations. The introspective psychology based on empiricism required consciousness to be analyzed into its elementary building blocks, the senseatoms. This introspective method required a strict separation between the observer's description of a datum of consciousness and the meaning of the observer about the datum. *Ebbinghaus'* invention of the nonsense syllables to be connected by external associations, and the behaviorist conception of stimulus-response units as 'behavioral atoms', may be seen as further manifestations of the empiricist philosophy (*Kvale*, 1975a).

The logical positivist methodology, tacitly adopted by most psychologists, was built on elementary logical atoms, corresponding to simple observational facts. The concept of a 'pure datum' is not a mere historical curiosity. *Russell* (1962) emphasized as the essential character of a datum that it is not inferred, it is a piece of knowledge that is not deducted. Recognizing the interpretative side to everyday perception, *Russell* (1962, p. 118) called for the reduction of interpretation in scientific methods: 'By these methods we can approach asymptotically to the pure datum. That there must be a pure datum is, I think, a logically irrefutable consequence of the fact that perception gives rise to new knowledge.' The contrary position of the line of positivism developed by *Mach* has had less impact on the conception of psychological methods. To *Mach*, facts are mainly theories to which we have become sufficiently accustomed (*Riegel*, 1975).

While the concepts of facts and data have been problematized in the philosophy of science, it is the naive concept of facts and data as 'in principle' free of interpretation which has prevailed in the common sense of the psychological community. The theoretical nature of psychological facts may be overlooked when the empiricist world outlook is taken for granted. The abstracting, isolating and quantifying approach to behavior no longer appears as one possible theoretical conception of psychology, but as the very scientific reflection of reality. To ask for the pure facts in psychology is therefore not a completely neutral methodological question, but may imply asking for an implicit empiricistic theory of behavior. The question we may put at this point is: when the request for more facts is made, what is then *not* asked for?

Dialectics

Dialectical thought, as developed by *Hegel* and further worked out by *Marx*, contrasts sharply with the metaphysical empiricist world outlook. From a dialectical perspective, the absolutizing of facts as the access to reality comes to give a distorted one-sided conception of human relations. Some main aspects of dialectics shall be outlined here, leaving out the divergencies between different dialectical traditions, as the purpose is to present a unitary conception to contrast to the empiricist facts-gathering.[1]

Dialectics involves studying human behavior as internally related to its *context*, emphasizing the social and historical aspects of the given situation.

[1] The following abbreviated and simplified presentation of dialectics is mainly based on the philosophical treatments by *Lukacs* (1971) and *Mao Tse-tung* (1968); and the applications to psychology by *Sartre* (1963), *Riegel* (1973), and *Wozniak* (1975).

Dialectics is the study of qualitative *changes* through the development of internal contradictions. The aim here is to grasp and conceptualize the stream of behavior, giving its change and stability due emphasis. In the process of becoming, something may both be and not be. The *status nascendi* has priority over the *status quo*.

Dialectics accepts *conflicting* and interdependent conceptions of a phenomenon.

Dialectics studies a phenomenon in its *internal* relations, involving aspects mutually implying and excluding each other. Internal contradictions within a phenomenon are the basis of development, which is influenced by external interrelations and interactions with other phenomena.

Dialectics is the study of the *qualitative* development of phenomena, of one quality changing into another. Quantitative increases may lead to qualitative changes. The focus is on qualitative transformations and radical breaks.

Dialectics emphasizes the *interdependence* of observing subject and the observed phenomenon, of observation and active interpretation. Men act upon the world, change it, and are again changed by the consequences of their actions.

Dialectics seeks the *essence* of a phenomenon. Immediate experience reveals a superficial surface level of reality, whereas the essence is only disclosed in the course of an extensive and concrete study of a phenomenon.

Dialectics is the *concrete* analysis of concrete conditions. In order to understand a phenomenon it must be investigated in its multiple aspects, i. e., its internal contradictions and relations to the social and historical context.

Dialectics does not accept the possibility of value-neutral descriptions and theories, but aims at accomplishing changes through *praxis*. The criterion of knowledge is the praxis it leads to.

This presentation might suggest the erroneous view of empiricism and dialectics as thesis and antithesis, requiring a synthesis encompassing the two poles. The antithesis of the empiricist focus on facts is, however, rationalism. Dialectics is itself a synthesis of empiricist observation and speculative rationalism through a descriptive and an interpretative approach to the phenomena, whereby the emphasis is on knowledge leading to action in a contradictory and developing world.

The writer holds that understanding human behavior demands a dialectical rationale, but such dialectics remains in psychology merely implicit and generally denied. The dialectical nature of qualitative methods in psychology has been pointed out by several authors, especially with respect to psychoanalytical therapy (e. g., *Fenichel*, 1970; *Reich*, 1929; *Rychlak*, 1968). In *The problem of Method, Sartre* (1963) demonstrates the necessity of phenomenological and dialectical qualitative methods in the social sciences. It would, however, be wrong to equate dialectics with 'soft' qualitative methods. *Marx*'s (1952) dialectical analysis of capitalism was based on historical descriptions as well as on economical statistics, working itself below the immediate manifestations of capitalism to uncover its essential contradictions and total developing tendencies.

The relative merits of quantitative and qualitative methods in psychology shall not be pursued here, nor the dialectical aspects of qualitative methods, which have often been dismissed as unscientific since they do not yield 'hard', objective facts (see Chapter 10). We shall instead argue the thesis of a dialectical foundation for scientific psychology by explicating the dialectical basis of the hard, quantifiable, data of psychology.

The Dialectics of Facts

Historically the concepts of data and facts came into language around the 16th Century. Although they are generally used synonymously today, data and facts are derived from different etymological roots. *Datum* means literally a *thing given* or granted – 'les données' in French. *Factum* means a *thing done* or performed. The German word for fact implies a thing done – 'Tatsache'. The Latin verb 'facere', to do, is the root of factum as well as of feat, manufacture, factory. Data are thus given, while facts are done, but both imply that something is observed as distinguished from speculation. Data and facts refer to things, not thoughts. Datum and factum are past participles, referring to the finished past, the 'passé defini' in French, that which may not change and develop.

By discussing the contradictions in the use of the data concept in psychology, its implicit dialectical basis may be brought out. Some important aspects of the empiricist and positivist conception of psychological data appear in a description by *Spence* (1956, p. 12) of *John Watson's* view of data:

> . . . the data of the psychologist are of exactly the same kind as those of the physical scientist. That is to say, immediate experience, the initial matrix out of which all sciences develop, is no longer to be conceived as the special province of psychology. The psychologist, like other natural scientists, simply must take consciousness for granted and proceed to his task of describing certain happenings occurring in it and discovering and formulating the nature of the relationships holding among them.

Data as given or inferred. The belief of *Watson* and *Spence* in data as immediately given, and of *Russell* in the existence of a 'pure datum', is opposed by several social scientists, who emphasize the theoretical presuppositions of facts. *Coombs* (1964, pp. 4–5) analyzed the processes by which data are made, concluding 'that the data are in part a product of the mind of the observer . . . all knowledge is the result of theory – we buy information with assumptions – "facts" are inferences, and so also are data and measurements and scales'. The naive taking of data for granted has also been contested within behaviorist methodology:

> The operation of auxiliary hypotheses in the expression of even the simplest protocol statement precludes any easy definition of 'fact' or 'datum'. It seems reasonable to conclude that the status of protocol statements in psychology can be properly assessed only when they are put in relation to a more extensive explanatory system (*Mandler and Kessen*, 1964, p. 191).

It seems clear that psychologists have not yet settled on a common view of 'the facts' which are so often alluded to in their scientific accounts. Today the terms data and facts are occasionally used synonymously, occasionally with contrasting meanings, e. g.: '. . . psychological facts depend on the interpretation of data' (*Deese*, 1972, p. 67) and 'The *fact* is the actual occurrence of the event; the *datum* is the recording of that event' (*McCain and Segal*, 1969, p. 32).

We regard the confusion in use of such terms as 'observation', 'fact', and 'datum' as due to the empiricist's false dichotomization of facts from theory, as well as the neglect of the constitution of data. The contradiction of supposed 'pure' or 'raw' facts and theoretical facts may be seen as the freezing of the dialectical relation between facts and theory, an absolutizing of one of the poles in the relation. In a dialectical view, there exists a reciprocal relation between facts and theory, both implying and excluding each other (*Kosik*, 1971).

Data as physical or mental. While the data concept is ambiguous with respect to its immediate givenness or theoretical nature, it is also ambiguous with respect to how the data of psychology are immediately given – i. e., as physical or mental. In early behaviorism, psychological data were conceived exactly the same as in the natural sciences. Thus, *Watson* (1935) required behavior to be described in strict physical terms without any reference to the meaning of behavior. Recently, an opposite position has been advocated; i. e., to consider *'meanings as data':* 'The meaning of what is said is experienced immediately by the observer and is therefore a primary datum . . . the raw data of psychology consist exclusively in the public meanings of the subject's acts' (*Smedslund*, 1969, pp. 5–8).

From a dialectical viewpoint, there is no reason to define psychological data as either physical *or* mental; they have their origin in the intentional behavior of a bodily subject in a material situation. The absolutizing of the bodily movements as physical, and the intentional directedness of behavior as mental, may be seen as representing the classical philosophical positions of mechanical materialism and idealism.

Trying to remain completely in the language realm of pure physical descriptions has not been easy for the behaviorist. In a critique of the 'behaviorist fallacy' – i. e., presuming that one is dealing in so-called objective behavior, operating completely independent of the observer – *From* (1971) documents how *Watson*, despite explicit efforts to the contrary, could not avoid referring to goals and intentions in his own descriptions of infant behavior.

An attitude common to much psychological observation was expressed by *Bales* (1951, p. 35). Scoring behavior in small groups to obtain objective data, he sought to balance between immediate experience and deeper interpretations of meaning, instructing the observers to 'work more or less on the surface meaning of activity and forego involved depth interpretations. The context which can be kept in mind is more or less confined to the "present" '. The requirement of strictly objective meaning data may imply a confinement to some 'mini-contexts' of the immediate present, where the appearance of the phenomena comes to take a scientific priority over their essential structures. A focus on surface meaning may be legitimate for certain scientific purposes, but, in a dialectical view, this is not more scientific than deeper, and possibly more controversial interpretations of the meaning of behavior.

While the strict physicalist conception of psychological data is seldom advocated today, the implicit *de facto* meaning basis of psychological data has remained theoretically unreflected in the mainstream tradition, while being analyzed in phenomenological approaches to psychology (*Skjervheim*, 1959; *Strasser*, 1963; *Giorgi*, 1970). The temporal and social perspectivity in the interpretation of meaning contrasts with the requirement of objective immutable and intersubjective data (*Kvale*, 1975b).

The immutability and intersubjectivity of data. The call for 'objective' data has been a cornerstone in the empiricist and positivist philosophy of science. Its objectivity criteria are expressed in two principles – *intra*subjective reproducibility: repeated observations of the same behavior by the same observer shall give the same data; *inter*subjective reproducibility: repeated observation of the same behavior by different observers shall give the same data (e. g., *Galtung*, 1967).

A strict enforcement of the criteria of intra- and inter-subjectively reproducible data may function as a methodological straightjacket, restricting a psychological science to rather superficial aspects of behavior, and to behavior which has become fixed and standardized, while the developing and controversial form of behavior is ruled out as unscientific.

In his historical study of scientific revolutions in physics, *Kuhn* (1962) came rather close to a dialectical – though idealistic – conception of science. He distinguished between 'normal' science within a stable and shared paradigm, and scientific crises in which the established paradigm is challenged by fundamentally new ways of doing and conceiving science. *Kuhn* here applied the analogy of ambiguous visual Gestalts, such as a figure which at one moment unequivocally appears as a duck, and in the next moment is just as certainly a rabbit. Such qualitative transformations, or Gestalt switches, create, even within physics, problems in the obtaining of intra- and intersubjectively reproducible data. As *Kuhn* (1962, p. 149) noted:

> Practicing in different worlds, the two groups of scientists see different things when they look from the same point in the same direction . . . That is why a law that cannot even be demonstrated to one group of scientists may occasionally seem intuitively obvious to another. Equally, it is why, before they can hope to communicate fully, one group or the other must experience the conversion that we have been calling a paradigm shift.

The possibility of acquiring immutable and uncontroversial data then appears limited to both phenomena and epochs in the development of a science characterized by relative stability and agreement. An absolutization of the strict demands of unequivocal, immutable and intersubjective data may hamper new breakthroughs in knowledge. In an evolving and conflicting human reality, it would be wrong to limit science to the apparently stable and uncontroversial surface of the social world. A dialectical approach emphasizes radical changes and conflicts as the important loci of acquiring knowledge, where the new tendencies, superseding the old, are breaking through to become real.

Facts and values. Within positivist philosophy of science the observed facts are to be strictly separated from values. To believe that facts are 'theory-laden' and yet maintain that facts are independent of values is contradictory. In a dialectical view, value-neutral descriptions are a theoretical impossibility because any description occurs within a given horizon of praxis. There is no pure knowledge upon which decisions can be based. Knowledge and action are two aspects of an original dialectical relation (cf. *Kvale and Grenness*, 1967). Our knowledge of the world is acquired through action upon the world; and the knowledge obtained thereby is again part of a broader encompassing activity.

Skinner (1961, 1974) is one of the few psychologists who dismisses the separation of facts and values, as well as the common criteria for objective data – 'exact reproducibility' and 'truth by agreement'. He acknowledges a technical interest of control, not only in the application of data, but also in their very constitution. To *Skinner* the essense of the description of behavior is to obtain data that show orderly changes. His criteria to behavioral data are consistency in obtaining successful operations upon the material studied; that is, the determination of orderliness of changes in the form of functional laws between stimulus and response. However, *Skinner*'s surpassing of the positivistic distinction of statements of facts and judgments of values remains limited to the field of technical action.

The constitution of facts. A strict line of demarcation between statements of facts and judgments of value can only be maintained as long as the observational behavior constituting the data is neglected. In a phenomenological approach to the social sciences, the surpassing of the 'repression' of the subjective constitution of objective data has been a central theme. In an analysis of the crisis of psychology, *Husserl* (1962) objected to the positivist reduction of the idea of science to a mere science of facts. He criticized the 'objectivist illusion' of taking the facts for granted, the belief of a reality-in-itself consisting of facts. *Merleau-Ponty* (1962) has further analyzed the 'prejudice of the objective world' – the conception of the world as a ready-made universe of facts. He acknowledged 'The whole universe of science is built upon the world as directly experienced', but, contrary to *Spence*, went on to state 'and if we want to subject science itself to rigorous scrutiny and arrive at a precise assessment of its meaning and scope, we must begin by reawakening the basic experience of the world of which science is the second-order expression' (*Merleau-Ponty*, 1962, p. viii).

Facts are not mere prejudices. The collection and ordering of facts may give an adequate picture of the manifest appearance of human interaction. The common methodological rules of facts-gathering and data analysis are fully legitimate on this level. But limiting a scientific psychology to the petrified facts also limits scientific knowledge to the surface structure of behavior, outlawing an analysis of the deeper, more essential contradictions of human behavior, and neglects the possibility of the immediate surface appearance of the phenomena concealing their essential structure.

The social consequences of the cult of facts were pointed out by *Husserl* (1962, p. 4): 'Blosse Tatsachenwissenschaften machen blosse Tatsachenmenschen'. *Habermas* (1971) has carried further *Husserl*'s critique of the 'objectivist illusion', emphasizing that when the constitution of facts is neglected, the insight into the interlocking of knowledge with interests from the life world is missed. *Habermas* postulates three fundamental knowledge interests, each constituting its subject matter – a technical interest in the natural sciences, a hermeneutic understanding interest in the humanistic sciences and a critical emancipatory interest in the social sciences. Thus, '. . . the facts relevant to the empirical sciences are first constituted through an a priori organisation of our experience in the behavioral system of instrumental action' (*Habermas*, 1971, p. 309). The observation that the 'interest in technical control over objectified processes' not only covers the application of data, but also constitutes how the data are given, has, with the exception of *Skinner*, generally been missed in most methodological treatments of the data of natural science psychology.

The Material Basis of Facts

Scientific facts are constituted by human activity in a material and social world, and they again influence the world as knowledge and ideology. Some aspects of this broader context of facts may be suggested by a historical perspective.

At a time when scholastics had ruled the universities, the development of the natural sciences was furthered by an empiricist philosophy basing knowledge on facts. The power of the natural sciences in acquiring systematic knowledge and control over natural processes was to a large degree a result of the movement from speculation to empirical observation. In the 17th Century, *Bacon's* requirement of observable data as the basis of knowledge also served the rising bourgeoisie in its conflict with the aristocratic feudal society. This stable and hierarchical society was legitimized by a theology, in which scholastic disputes rested on the interpretation of the scriptures by the learned few, as well as on the presumed mystical intuitions of the occasional saint. Baconian appeals to basic knowledge in facts, which in principle were open to the observation of everyone, represented a progressive accomplishment of the historical period. The trend to depersonalize knowledge, to make it common and intersubjective, was in contrast to the personal authority of a restricted group of scholars, and to the personal rule of a king and noble class. Knowledge based on facts became a power of the bourgeoisie in its conflict with the theologically legitimized aristocracy.

Also the 19th Century positivism was to serve the bourgeoisie, according to the explicit intentions of *Comte*, by protecting their privileges and securing their domination of the rising working class (*Samelson*, 1974). In contrast to *J. S. Mill* and most later positivists, *Comte* emphasized the inherent unity of the positivist methodology and the system of positive politics. His 'Sociocracy' was to be ruled by industrialists and bankers, and the proletariat kept in its place without striving for more than was their due by a positivist scientist-priesthood. Their main function besides guiding public opinion was education, which was to make the supervision of the workers more effective. Referring to the growing interest for his positivism in the United States, *Comte* (1902, p. 48; cited in *Samelson*, 1974, p. 227) wrote '. . . one senses already that the family and property can be defended only by a new spiritual power . . . our *yankee* friends now envisage *Positivism* as alone able to save them from communism'.

In the same period as *Comte* (1798–1857) was advocating positivism as the bourgeoisie's ideology for dominating the working class, *Marx* (1818–1883), by his materialist transformation of *Hegel*'s dialectics, developed dialectical materialism. It was not conceived as an ahistorical or universal method, but as determined by the nature of the phenomena to be analyzed. Dialectical materialism was to acquire scientific knowledge of the contradictions and oppression of the capitalist society. Serving the rising working class it was both a method of cognizing reality and an instrument of the revolutionary remaking of the world. The contradictions in men's thinking and action were to be traced to the contradictions in the material basis of society.

From a dialectical materialist viewpoint, the empiricist and positivist philosophy is considered not only as furthering knowledge, but also as reflecting the material and social contradictions of a certain epoch, and, at the same time, functioning ideologically to conceal insight into these contradictions. Thus, according to *Mao Tse-tung* (1968), the metaphysical, empiricist world outlook suppresses the dialectical insight that society contains within its very structure a series of contradictions, working themselves forward, transforming the society which is ever mobile and not the rigid *status quo* which the metaphysical empiricism makes it out to be.

Lukacs (1971) has addressed himself more specifically to the reifying function of facts in bourgeois ideology. He derived the concept of reified consciousness from *Marx*'s analysis of industrial production and exchange of commodities under capitalism, where essentially socially determined human relations are presented in the disguised appearance as relations between things. The products of human activity appear in the reified consciousness as something objective, and independent of human activity. In the bourgeois sciences' fetishization of the fact, the reified structure of the human world under capitalism comes to appear as the only scientific reality possible. The observed human behavior is captured in a web of rational calculation as reified, fixed and isolated data. These sciences form facts of the immediately given reality, concealing the historical and social character of such facts, whose essential nature rests on human relationships. It is only by breaking the methodological priority of facts that the nature of a phenomenon as process can be grasped:

> Only then will it be understood that the facts are nothing but the parts, the *aspects* of the total process that have been broken off, artificially isolated and ossified . . . it also becomes clear why in the reified thought of the bourgeoisie in the 'facts' have to play the part of its highest fetish in both theory and practice. This petrified factuality in which everything is frozen into a 'fixed magnitude', in which the reality that just happens to exist persists in a totally senseless, unchanging way precludes any theory that could throw light on even this immediate reality (*Lukacs*, 1971, p. 184).

The material basis of knowledge is subject to historical change. The transition in the forces of production from handicrafts to industrial manufacture involved an elimination of the qualitative human factor, where the previous unitary work process was fragmented into isolated operations. The industrial division of labor entailed a separation of manual and mental labor, the production process became mechanized and the control and planning transferred to the management. The factual issue of carrying out the production was left to the workers, while the issue of values, of deciding what ought to be produced, was the task of the management. The exact quantification and calculation of the atomized work operations was at the end of the 19th Century made into a science of 'human engineering' by *Taylor*'s time-and-motion studies. Shortly thereafter, the fragmentation of the work process into externally connected elements was perfected by the assembly line introduced by *Ford*.

The mechanical fragmentation of the process of production may be reflected in the mechanistic atomization of knowledge into isolated facts. The division between manual and mental labor may have provided a basis for the physicalist and mentalist conceptions of behavior (*Rubinsteijn*, 1963) and of psychological data. And the separation of workers and management may relate to the dichotomization of facts and values. The technological standardization of society may have furthered the conception of knowledge as based on immutable and intersubjective objective data.

The technologizing of manual and mental operations is gradually providing a pervasive structure of 'the technological society' (*Ellul*, 1964). Technology implies breaking down the previously integrated human process of production into its smallest elements, and treating them as raw material to be mechanically connected into new units. The so-called knowledge industry processes vast amounts of information about human behavior, where the objective and isolated data function as raw material, to be conjoined through externally programmed patterns. The relating of the empiricist data cult to industrial technology is not a mere analogy. Today we witness a synthesis of the two in the expanding industry of *data technology* (*Kvale*, 1975b).

The development of technology is not unequivocal. There is today a trend away from the conception of immutable and isolated data as finished products to a focus on processes and qualitative transformations (*Toffler*, 1971). If such trends in current technology develop further, some of the material basis for the psychological fetishization of facts might wane.

Some Closing Observations

The ambiguities and contradictions of the psychological fact concept are not due to mere scientific immaturity or weakness, but may be traced to the contradictions of a capitalist technological society. The general reification of consciousness through the forces and relations of production in capitalism, whereby the products of human activity appear in the form of objectively given things, may also provide a frame of reference for the positivist conception of facts objectively and immediately given, independent of the observer. According to *Adorno* (1970), the truth of positivism is that only in an unfree society have the facts as given taken on impenetrable power, which is then duplicated in scientific thought as the 'cult of facts'.

Few social scientists would today adhere to *Comte*'s intentions of subduing the workers through positivism. Nevertheless, there may be oppressive social consequences of the current myth of facts. The data constituted through the technical interest in control over objectified processes freezes a technological approach to human reality as the only scientific reality. The definition of the social reality becomes a matter for social engineers and scientists, whereby the participants' own definition of their world becomes secondary to the technologically constituted reality. The scientific value placed on impersonal knowledge in the form of objective facts may facilitate adaptation to modern methods of domination. Oppression occurs today less through direct personal domination, than by anonymous bureaucratic and technological means – primarily through the supposedly 'objective', nature-given forms of economic exploitation. As human interaction is increasingly taking the form of reified economical relations and technological structures, the scientific focus on objective facts is becoming a more and more adequate representation of the surface appearance of a capitalist society, while at the same time concealing its essential nature, as resting on oppressive human relations.

References

Adorno, T. W.: Aufsätze zur Gesellschaftstheorie und Methodologie (Suhrkamp, Frankfurt 1970).

Bales, R. F.: Interaction process analysis (Addison-Wesley, Cambridge 1951).

Comte, A.: Lettres d'Auguste Comte à divers, vol. I. (Fonds Typographique, Paris 1902).

Coombs, C. H.: A theory of data (Wiley, New York 1964).

Deese, J.: Psychology as science and art (Harcourt, Brace, Jovanovich, New York 1972).

Ellul, J.: The technological society (Vintage, New York 1964).

Fenichel, O.: Über die Psychoanalyse als Keim einer zukünftigen dialektisch-materialistischen Psychologie; in Marxismus, Psychoanalyse, Sexpol 1, pp. 229–249 (Fischer, Frankfurt 1970).

From, F.: Perception of other people (Columbia University Press, New York 1971).

Galtung, J.: Theory and methods of social research (Universitetsforlaget, Oslo 1967).

Giorgi, A.: Psychology as a human science (Harper & Row, New York 1970).

Goethe, J. W.: Maximen und Reflexionen (Verlag der Goethe-Gesellschaft, Weimar 1907).

Habermas, J.: Knowledge and human interests (Beacon, Boston 1971).

Husserl, E.: Die Krisis der europäischen Wissenschaften und die transzendentale Phänomenologie (Nijhoff, Den Haag 1962).

Kosik, K.: Dialektik des Konkreten (Suhrkamp, Frankfurt 1971).

Kuhn, T. S.: The structure of scientific revolutions (Chicago University Press, Chicago 1962).

Kvale, S.: Memory and dialectics: some reflections on Ebbinghaus and Mao Tse-tung. Hum. Dev. *18* (in press, 1975a).

Kvale, S.: Meanings as data and human technology (Unpublished, University of Aarhus, 1975b).

Kvale, S. and Grenness, C. E.: Skinner and Sartre: towards a radical phenomenology of behavior? Rev. existent. Psychol. Psychiat. *7:* 128–150 (1967).

Lukacs, G.: History and class consciousness (Merlin, London 1971).

Mandler, G. and Kessen, W.: The language of psychology (Wiley, New York 1964).

Mao Tse-tung: Four essays on philosophy (Foreign Languages Press, Peking 1968).

Marx, K.: in *Hutchins* Great books of the western world, vol. 50, p. 1–393 (Encyclopedia Britannica, Chicago 1952).

McCain, G. and Segal, E. M.: The game of science (Brooks/Cole, Belmont 1969).

Merleau-Ponty, M.: Phenomenology of perception (Routledge Kegan / Humanities Press, London/New York 1962).

Reich, W.: Dialektischer Materialismus und Psychoanalyse. Unter dem Banner des Marxismus (1929).

Riegel, K. F.: Introduction to developmental and historical structuralism; in *Riegel and Rosenwald* Structure and transformation; developmental and historical aspects, p. 36–57 (Wiley, New York 1975).

Rubinsteijn, S. L.: Prinzipien und Wege der Psychologie (Akademie-Verlag, Berlin 1963).

Russell, B.: An inquiry into meaning and truth (Penguin, Harmondsworth 1962).

Rychlak, J. F.: A philosophy of science for personality theory (Houghton Mifflin, Boston 1968).

Samelson, F.: History, origin, myth and ideology: 'discovery' of social psychology. J. Theory soc. Behav. *4:* 217–231 (1974).

Sartre, J.-P.: The problem of method (Methuen, London 1963).

Skinner, B. F.: Cumulative record (Appleton, Century Crofts, New York 1961).

Skinner, B. F.: About behaviorism (Knopf, New York 1974).

Skjervheim, H.: Objectivism and the study of man (Universitetsforlaget, Oslo 1959).

Smedslund, J.: Meanings, implications and universals: towards a psychology of man. Scand. J. Psychol. *10:* 1–15 (1969).

Spence, K. W.: Behavior theroy and conditioning (Yale University Press, New Haven 1956).

Strasser, S.: Phenomenology and the human sciences (Duquesne University Press, Pittsburgh 1963).

Toffler, A.: Future shock (Random House, New York 1971).

Watson, J. B.: Psychology as a natural science. The failure of psychology as a mental science; in *Skinner* Readings in psychology, p. 809–811 (Holt, Rinehart & Winston, New York 1935).

Wozniak, R. H.: Dialecticism and structuralism in Soviet philosophy and psychology; in *Riegel and Rosenwald* Structure and transformation: developmental and historical aspects (Wiley, New York 1975, in press).

Contr. hum. Dev., vol. 2, pp. 101–112 (Karger, Basel 1976)

Chapter 10
The Dialectic and Qualitative Methodology

Susan V. Lourenço

Introduction

The behavioral sciences set out to study the complexities and realities of human behavior. More often than not, however, the methods of explanation by which social scientists attempt to characterize social events tend to remove them from the very phenomena they wish to study. On the one hand, we have the tradition whereby human behavior is approached via a natural science model. This 'empirical' tradition, in which much research in psychology and sociology has been conducted in the last 50 years, is 'absolutistic, outer-directed and intolerant of ambiguity' (*Kagan*, 1967, p. 131). On the other hand, we have the tradition of 'verstehen', derived from *Weber*, where the methodology is more likely to be qualitative than quantitative. Such a perspective 'assumes that understanding can only be achieved by actively participating in the life of the observed and gaining insight by means of introspection' (*Bruyn*, 1963, p. 229).

The social sciences have been slower than the physical sciences to legitimately admit of doubt, uncertainty, antithesis, and paradox. Qualitative studies have, more often than not, been regarded with disdain or as not admitting of 'scientific' or 'hard' scholarship. Defined, qualitative methodology is that strategy of investigation which allows the researcher to participate in the social phenomena being studied. Field work, participant observation, and in-depth interviewing together form a set of techniques to gather, record, verify and analyze data collected about human beings in their natural settings. The investigator's own humanity is not forgotten, in that he, or she, not only gets close to the data, but admittedly becomes a part of it and thus a part of the analysis. If the needs of the investigator are to become a part of the social process of research while he or she *also* remains an outsider, or a 'scientist', then resulting tensions and conflicts may be anticipated. It is these conflicts that have not been formally examined in studies employing qualitative methodology. In the present chapter, the author suggests that qualitative methodology, in itself, is imbued with a dialectic which the researcher employing these methods should perhaps be aware of.

In qualitative methodology, the investigator is not only sensitive to the usual factors influencing the dependent variables under study, but develops a dialectical self-consciousness regarding how he or she as a conceptualizer or a 'person', may be influencing the course of inquiry. One's attitude toward the subject-object dichotomy is more sophisticated in such an approach (see *Dewey and Bentley*, 1954). There is concrete evidence that rigid distinctions between what is subjective and what is completely objective cannot be maintained in research on human beings (e. g., *Dexter*, 1970; *Friedman*, 1967; *Rosenthal*, 1966). Even so, as already noted, the physical sciences today are more accepting of a lessened bifurcation between subjective and objective than are the social sciences. The necessary and continuing dialectic between the role of 'member' (participant in the system) and 'stranger' (observer, reporter, scientist) is what all researchers in field work have in common (*Hughes*, 1960, p. xi).

A second role for dialectic in the present chapter will be found in the fact that it is readily seen functioning as an active principle in social life. Most scholars admit of a role for dialectic in the realm of logic, as if it were something employed only in the more abstract realms of thought – often as a kind of illogic or 'sophistry' (see Chapter 1). But the investigator who approaches field work with an appreciation of dialectical reasoning cannot fail to see its operation in the mundane activities of everyday life. As *Pribram* (1949, p. 3) has observed, in the dialectical pattern of thought is found the 'ability to interpret all phenomena and events because of their continuously changing aspects'. The dialectic 'allows one to pose problems overlooked or minimized by social scientists which do not take account of the continuous transformation in social relationships' (*Haldane*, 1938, p. 155). Dialectical thought has been aptly termed 'the perception of existential contradiction' (*Murphy*, 1971, p. 229). If human beings *are* existentially contradictory and continuously undergoing a process of change, how else is it possible for the social scientist to conceptualize and understand their behavior but through the heuristic benefits of a dialectical construct?

The present chapter is devoted to a discussion of the qualitative methodology employed by the writer in studying a large commercial television station for 2 years (*Lourenço*, 1974). She assumed the role of a participant observer and came to see all aspects of this business organization 'from the inside'. A major focus of the study had to do with social conflicts, i. e., the problems of managing the station, of working within it, and with the consequent tensions which arose in day-to-day interactions. No attempt will be made to summarize the many findings of this investigation. In the present context, we hope merely to discuss the question of qualitative methodology, in an effort to give the reader some idea of what is meant by this phrase as well as the reasons for seeking an alternative to the classical 'quantitative' methodology now being practiced in the social sciences.

Participant observation, or the study of a social system by interactive observation, has been said to involve 'taking account of the socio-cultural world – the complex of actors and their plot as they live and dream on the stage of society' (*Bruyn*, 1966, p. xxiv). Complex interactions and events were therefore studied by the writer as they actually happened, with the only intrusion being that she was called upon at times to make recommendations having a formative influence on the very data she was observing. A major premise understood from the beginning of the field work was that only a critical comprehension of present reality can precede active intervention in a social system. Data were obtained in a variety of forms – e. g., documents, observations, informal interviews – and concerned the day-to-day life, interactions, and culture of a modern organization. Written notes were taken on the spot, reviewed, and expanded within a day or two before being typed in final form. The television station's documents and formal records were also analyzed, as were memoranda and correspondence (unless restrictions were put on such data; refer below). Much of the data collected were 'unobtrusive' (*Webb et al.*, 1966), i. e., taken from routine sources rather than produced merely for the purposes of this study.

How the Dialectic Helped

In an absolute sense, conflicts are never solved by the dialectic. But in a relative sense, they are 'being solved'. The sequential discussion begins again around a new point, which subsumes or takes account of the 'best' that has gone before. A dialectical conceptualization was useful at several stages of the research process: as noted above, in helping to understand the initial problem; in the desire to construe the reality and meanings of social life while adhering to canons of scientific scholarship; in clarifying the types of ambiguities or conflicting impressions gleaned on first entering the organization; in defining the writer's role of researcher vis-à-vis the subjects at various points in time and at various levels of the organization; and, in analyzing and interpreting the data during and after its collection.

In the discussion to follow, an account is given of some of the problems confronting a participant observer in an organization. The focus is on data collection, analysis, and interpretation. Examples of the dialectic are used throughout to illustrate factors involved in the conduct of the study and in its interpretation. Lastly, the dialectic is employed heuristically to clarify the researcher's role during the field observations as well as the theoretical commentary which followed.

Entry

The problems associated with 'entry' in field research and the need for a target system and an observer to establish value-congruence and complementation in regard to role are well known (*Glidewell,* 1959). Entry may involve resorting to a 'mechanism of defense, a defense against his [consultant's or observer's] own uncertainty and against the ambiguities of the situation' (*Vansina,* 1970). The observer's values and goals may be on one side, the organization's values and goals on the other (thesis and antithesis). For example, in the study being depicted, the writer initially had little knowledge about the world of communications and none at all about the world of television. She had never been associated with business in the role of researcher. Her own assumptions and understandings were minimal, as were those of the organization regarding her role in carrying out observations. Initially, she was introduced to a group of managers. The group was told only that she wanted to study the organization 'as a whole', and that she wanted also to understand the lives of people working in the television station. Nothing was said regarding the researcher's interest in social conflict, conflict resolution or the dialectic. Initial expectations were set up concerning the observer's role; i. e., observation at the option of the persons involved and informal interviewing of participating subjects. Entry into the organization's culture bore few problems and was eased in that the bridge to the organization was via an executive whose status was anything but marginal. This executive, if not a 'Doc' (*Whyte*, 1955), was certainly a cooperative gatekeeper and a great support to the observer.

First Impressions

In the beginning, it was important to understand social behavior within the overall cultural setting of the organization. Thus, learning about television operations, the language of sales and technology, and the commercial and artistic nature of the television industry had to be comprehended, if not thoroughly understood. At the same time, certain fears of individuals had to be alleviated. Few people had ever encountered a researcher whose interest was in human relations rather than in learning about broadcasting or television *per se*. Some were afraid that the observer was interested in their personalities. Others voiced an initial fear that she was a 'spy' from the company headquarters. Clearly, the subjective, human dimension was always present in the work. When both subject matter and observer are human, relations between the two cannot be ignored. Moreover, the relationship is imbued with both tension and conflict.

It proved helpful to view the problem of entry, first impressions, and the formation of a role for the observer as a conflict involving two 'moments' in the dialectic. The expectations and accommodations worked out between the observer and the organization had to be negotiated in such a way that both parties received something from the interchange which was perceived as equitable. Since the norm of reciprocity upon which this notion is based is unstable, the same cycle of negotiation continued often and at different levels within the organization (*Gouldner*, 1960). Yet, the structure of the conflict is always the same: a thesis on the one side, an antithesis on the other. Accommodations between observer and organization are begun at new points and are based on the increasing knowledge each side has of the other via the previous negotiations.

Role of the Observer

The problem of learning to be an observer, said *Hughes*, is like the 'problem of learning to live in society' (*Hughes*, 1960, p. xv). Expectations and accommodations had to be worked out between the organization and the observer in such a way that both parties received something from the interchange, and so that both perceived the return to be equitable. This can prove a difficult job, especially when the observer, as in the present instance, learned that certain managers expected her to comment and make recommendations on 'managerial style'. She had not anticipated taking on the role of a process consultant, but it was natural in listening and observing to absorb a great deal of useful information concerning how a part of the organization was being administered. Indeed, there was also a natural inclination to be drawn to those who sought feedback regarding their managerial style, since this helped to validate the observer as a knowledgeable person. The observer found that she had to guard against a one-sided perspective of the organization in this sense. Despite the reward of feeling she was perhaps contributing something to the people in the organization, providing feedback made the observer feel uncomfortable. She failed to analyze this discomfort, and instead reiterated her 'observer' role to the participants in what probably came across properly as a 'lame excuse'. This, more likely than not, resulted in a perception of inequity on the part of the subjects toward the observer.

The dilemma of wanting to collect data and share insights once gathered, while at the same time not betraying professional standards of disinterested objectivity was resolved by withdrawing from the organization and essentially standing back from it. The level of marginality thus achieved was varied as time went by. Interviews were conducted out of the work context to some extent, and gradually a greater understanding of the total organization was gained by the observer. One great advantage which the observer had was that she could do more of such *interrelating* of factors than even the managers of the organization could. Since there are both visible and invisible factors involved in human relations, by having access to certain attitudes, to the 'looks' of people interviewed or to cues given when certain issues were raised, etc., it was possible to return to the everyday organizational context with more understanding than any single person in the totality. The observer found that without some such total overview, the dynamics of the television station could not be fully understood. As the observer learned more about different aspects and levels of the organization, she took greater risks and reduced her marginality once again. The following abstract from the field notes illustrates this point:

> Fred, an engineer, complains about bad communication in the organization: 'People hear about things circuitously, and that's bad. More than that, there's a feeling you can't advance. There aren't many rewards, but there aren't many criticisms either.' I (observer) understand this to mean that the organizational life is 'flat', with no real highs or lows. Yet, some of my other data do not confirm this picture. I bring up the station's 'discrepancy reports', in which the critiques of employee performance are generally detailed and even quite severe. 'Oh yeah', drawls Fred. 'I feel like a jury "trying" a drunken driver, knowing all the while 'it could've been me.' He goes on to discuss the responsibility of having to write such reports, and to make the very 'high and low' decision points which he seemed to imply were not the case earlier in our interview.

Although this interchange might be seen as the observer simply asking for further clarification in cross-checking her information, in point of fact it was a calculated dialectical confrontation in which the observer purposively searched her materials with an eye to possible inconsistencies. Doubtless this occurs spontaneously in field work, where a researcher employs dialectical strategies unawares. But the point of the present chapter is to show that there *is* a specific qualitative methodology at play in such encounters, and that it can be cultivated to the profit of the study being conducted.

The dialectic also helped in generating descriptive concepts and explanations of what had been observed. Watching people at work in an organization brought many activities under the rubric of, e. g., positive/negative, stability/change, or conservative/revolutionary insofar as events could be conceptualized. For example, a conflict which arose in the television station over personnel policies was helpfully viewed as one involving conservative versus revolutionary features. Since the synthesis involved a redefinition of the standardized roles for men and women as well as blacks and whites, the resolution of this conflict was not forthcoming. Possibly, had the poles of opposition been construed as less disparate, a resolution would have been forthcoming, but the two sides seemed unable to redefine their stand vis-à-vis relations between the sexes or among the races.

Insofar as such explanations are concerned, we witness here a peculiarly human characteristic, a form of understanding or explanation of the 'facts' which freezes us into reality in one sense, but which can be reoriented thanks to the dialectical side of human reason. Explanations refer to the manner in which events or interactions can be predicted, based on an explicit set of observations that can be repeated by someone else. Insofar as the dialectic is concerned, it cannot be said to explain in this particular sense. *Findlay* (1958, p. 149) points out that synthesis cannot be deduced, so that *Hegel*'s 'dialectical ladder of notions has little in common with a deductive chain of propositions following one another according to fixed principles laid down in advance'. Thus, the dialectic cannot be used for prediction. Descriptive solutions are reached in dialectical analysis by a reinterpretation of the circumstances in light of a wider relation ('one in many'), given that the consensual starting point for a dialectic explanation is the existence of conflict. Once a dialectical course is predictable it is no longer truly dialectical!

The dialectic is thus more useful in creating knowledge than it is in explaining it. In a study of the process of perception and reasoning, *Abercrombie* (1960) demonstrated how students perceive by making them introspect in dialectical fashion – i. e., see both what they had and they had *not* seen. This led to more accurate perception. In other words, the notion of examining what is, tends to create what 'might be', or, in the quest for knowledge, 'there must always be a dynamic movement in verification, one that points to the "negative" elements latent in the current reality' (*Jay*, 1973, p. 82). The power of the intellect may therefore be used to create meanings from the raw data – as in the case cited above, by way of the field notes. It does not seem extreme to state that when the dialectic is viewed as a tool for the creation of data as well as descriptions of these data in a conceptual sense, it is at work 'in the mind'. This is invariably what we mean by the mind construct, insofar as we think of this as a contributory agent in existence.

The Dialectic and the Pursuit of Knowledge

Implied in the dialectic of knowledge-seeking is the notion of process and development, of interplay and the resolution of contradictions. Included here, too, is the notion that the 'sincerity and authenticity' (*Trilling*, 1972) of the social scientist are crucial ingredients to any understanding. The significance, therefore, of who the researcher is, what she did in the study described in this chapter, and how the data were interpreted lies not in the certainty of the presentation nor in the possibility of attaining absolute knowledge, but in the very contradictions which may be contained therein, and in the recognition that the social scientist plays an active role in creating this knowledge. In interacting both with the people in the organization at the time of the observations and with the data at the time of the writing (and rewriting) of the study, the dialectic allowed for the creation of a reciprocal relationship by which a perspective was attained, but not an absolute truth.

Nevertheless, the salient concerns of scientific scholarship were taken into account. Validity and reliability, degree of involvement, sampling, etc. were concerns that had to be met, albeit in nontraditional ways. A brief overview is followed by a more detailed discussion of some of these concerns.

The 'Participant' Aspect of Participant Observation

The 'participant' part of the observer role was limited in the present study, but involved the expression of some opinions, advice and suggestions concerning organizational problems. Observations were made of people at work. Sometimes an individual was followed through his or her daily work routine. At other times, all the people involved in certain settings were observed; e. g., staff meetings, mobile news crews, labor-management negotiations, or problem-solving conferences. At the outset, such persons and settings were selected on advice from management; after a few months of experience, observations were planned and made to insure coverage of representative settings and specific people in the quest of needed information. To increase trust and to reduce censuring of information, social distance between observer and observed was occasionally reduced. To gain perspective and control personal involvement, this social distance was occasionally increased. Finally, the recorded observations, interviews and content analyses of documents were reviewed, rearranged, analyzed and interpreted, with new understandings developing throughout the run of the study.

Along the way, however, there were pitfalls due to the fact that research in a natural setting is so personal in nature (*Whyte*, 1955, p. 279). The observer must avoid what *Devereux* (1967) calls 'counter-observation', particularly as regards the level of rapport achieved with the human beings functioning within the organization under study. One problem is that of under-rapport, which refers to the failure on the part of an observer to establish a reciprocity in the relationship with subjects under observation, so that relevant situations are not made available for observation. The writer's relationship with the television station's chief executive was typified by such under-rapport. He was the only person in the organization who excluded the writer from certain meetings or relevant work settings. Viewed in terms of the dialectic, the values of the researcher (thesis) and the subject (antithesis) never confronted each other in open dialogue so that a satisfactory synthesis might have been achieved. In such circumstances the researcher must look elsewhere for material, and thanks to the unity of any organizational totality (the 'one' among many) it is possible to fit the pieces together in a satisfactory manner.

The reverse problem is that of over-rapport, which refers to an excess of empathy for the organization and its members, as well as a tendency to identify oneself as part of the group under study to the detriment of marginality or objectivity (*Bruyn*, 1963). This is in some ways more difficult for the observer to deal with than under-rapport, for the behavioral scientist must come to terms with personal feelings and inclinations which are very threatening. In a two-person confrontation there is always the luxury of assigning partial responsibility to 'the other'. But in a case of over-rapport in the field research, the confrontation must be with one's self, meaning there is no leeway for rationalization or for the assigning of responsiblility to some incalcitrant subject under observation (*Sandler*, 1973). Working in a colorful industry like television, there was an obvious temptation for the observer 'to go native'. In fact, people told her at one point that she was being swept up by the 'glamour of show biz', and when she eventually accepted an academic appointment rather than a position in television, there were expressions of astonishment and disbelief. However, by dialectically confronting her motivations at various points throughout the study, the writer managed to keep her perspective and checked this tendency for overrapport with the television industry. Traditional discussions of participant observation do not cover this – very human – side to the work of the behavioral scientist, but obviously this is an unjustified oversight.

Reliability, Validity, and the Meaning of Research Findings

An implicit assumption of the study conducted was that the social forces at play in an organization are best understood if experienced and reacted to by someone actually living in the same social context. Since the study focused on social conflicts and their resolution, a natural strategy for description and illustration could be used without deteriorating into a tactic of persuasion. Illustration contains an inherent danger. It can be used as a means of persuasion, to give convincing evidence that things are indeed so. The dialectic method was a particularly useful way of countering this, in that (1) negative instances were sought and used illustratively as a matter of course, (2) exceptions to the rule were dealt with as legitimate instances rather than as error variance, and (3) alternative interpretations of the data were always offered. Since the research focused on a process, the methodology employed also stressed a process conception of the 'data' accrued.

These data have reliability and validity, but in employing qualitative methodology, we need to have a slightly different outlook on the nature of these traditional indicants. Qualitative research is sensitive to the descriptive terminology which a social environment – in this case, the television station – evolves in order to function. The task of participant observer is to understand and thereby identify the specific conceptual language, and to prove through analysis of critical incidents that the concepts so expressed *are* commonly understood and therefore *have* relevance to the functioning of the social unit. If the observer brings in new terminology to describe events taking place in the sociocultural world of its actors, then it must be shown how these meanings are being reflected in the everyday language of the group under study. This is a variant form of 'operational definition', whereby the target social unit is shown to have spontaneously reflected some more technical formulation in its everyday functioning.

For example, an observer may frame the problems faced by an individual in adjusting to the social demands of an organization in terms of a 'dominance-submission' construct dimension. Validity is established only if this terminology can be operationalized by giving illustrations of the activity in concrete instances. The subjects under observation need not refer to their adjustment problems in terms of dominance-submission. So long as the meaningful referents which may vary are demonstrably subsumed by the construct dimension, a reliability may be said to be seen taking place within the group. *Reliability* is therefore a general level of understanding concerning some conception in the organization as a whole. There is also the classical notion of reliability whereby two or more observers agree on the meaning being employed in describing the functioning of a group. In the case of participant observation, the former reliability is far more important than the latter, which is actually fairly easy to achieve. *Validity* arises from the demonstrable functioning of the meanings selected. Valid constructs 'make a difference' in the field study. If dominance and submission prove to be clarifying descriptive terms in several instances, we have attained a properly valid construct dimension – valid for *this* social unit and likely to be reflected in various guises.

This would hold true even if the experimenter were to give the same behavioral pattern a 'dominant' and then subsequently a 'submissive' interpretation. The validity does not lie in what 'is' the case for all time, but rather in the validity of the conceptualization being applied descriptively. In this sense, validity is closely tied to the meaning of a construct – as used by the observer, but also as used by the subjects under observation. Reliability takes us into the question of several persons understanding what is being expressed. The fundamental difference between this qualitative and the usual quantitative approach to reliability and validity is that what is being held up as data are the *bipolar meanings* of the scientist's descriptive terms – their general understanding and the utility they have as graphic labels for the descriptions being propounded – rather than the supposed *reality* of the unipolar designations as to what 'is' and what 'is not' taking place in observation. This is why it is so important to give both positive and negative instances, alternative explanations, exceptions to the rule, etc., in framing one's expository accounts.

Concluding Observations

The writer gave several talks to members of the organization and circulated preliminary drafts of the manuscript. Although the observations were generally agreed with, there was a noticeable reluctance to accept the existence of conflicts in the television station. This seems to be a general societal phenomenon, for in our culture interpersonal tensions are recognized only grudgingly, especially in a work setting where participants consider themselves to be 'on the same team'. It was also clear that dialectical thinking was alien to members of the organization. Not only is the structure of an organization ill-suited to the acceptance of critical thinking, but the positivistic climate of the American culture in general is ill-suited to an appreciation of the dialectic in human relations. The consumers of research, be they colleagues in universities or members of an organization, prefer to hear about absolute (unipolar) results rather than relative (multipolar) findings. There is great resistance to the use of doubt and alternative, or of conflict-laden descriptions. Anyone working in a dialectical frame must, therefore, anticipate a good deal of rejection from the average 'research public'.

In closing, the value of the dialectic as a metaconstruct (*Rychlak*, 1968), as an intellectual process in the execution and analysis of a qualitative study of the type discussed above, is not only of immense importance as a methodology, but also aids the development of an understanding of the social-scientific mode of inquiry in general. Moreover, if the behavioral sciences are going to provide fresh insights into social reality and the manner in which human beings, researchers and subjects alike, relate to this reality, then our present natural-science methods of study must be supplemented and in certain cases replaced by a methodology which is more representative of the social world we all recognize in our daily environments. No other method can capture the humanity of this social world more accurately than a dialectical method, one which provides the necessary interactive and in-depth analysis of both the data and the process, whereby such data are delineated through inquiry.

Reference

Abercrombie, M. L. J.: The anatomy of judgment: an investigation into the process of perception and reasoning (Hutchinson, London 1960).

Bloom, B. S. (ed.): Taxonomy of educational objectives; in Handbook I: cognitive domain (McKay, New York 1956).

Bruyn, S. T.: The methodology of participant observation. Hum. Org. *22:* 224–235 (1963).

Bruyn, S. T.: The human perspective in sociology: the methodology of participant observation (Prentice Hall, Englewood Cliffs 1966).

Devereux, G.: From anxiety to method in behavioral research (Mouton, The Hague, 1967).

Dewey, J. and Bentley, A. F.: Knowing and the known (Beacon, Boston 1954).

Dexter, L. A.: Elite and specialized interviewing (Northwestern University Press, Evanston 1970).

Findlay, J. N.: The philosophy of Hegel: an introduction and re-examination. (Collier, New York 1958).

Friedmann, N.: The social nature of psychological research (Basic Books, New York 1967).

Glidewell, J. C.: The entry problem in consultation. J. soc. Issues *15:* 51–60 (1959).

Gouldner, A. W.: The norm of reciprocity. Am. sociol. Rev. *25:* 161–179 (1960).

Haldane, J. B. S.: The Marxist philosophy and the sciences (Allen & Unwin, London 1938).

Hughes, E. C.: Introduction; in *Junker* An introduction to the social sciences pp. iii–xiii (University of Chicago Press, Chicago 1960).

Jay, M.: The dialectical imagination (Little, Brown, Boston 1973).

Kagan, J.: On the need for relativism. Am. Psychol. *22:* 131–142 (1967).

Lourenço, S. V.: Social conflict resolution and the dialectic; unpublished diss., University of Chicago, Chicago (1974).

Murphy, R. E.: The dialectic of social life: alarms and excursions in anthropological theory (Basic Books, New York 1971).

Pribram, K.: Conflicting patterns of thought (Washington Public Affairs Press, Washington 1949).

Rosenthal, R.: Experimenter effects in behavioral research (Appleton Century Crofts, New York 1966).

Rychlak, J. F.: A philosophy of science for personality theory (Houghton Mifflin, Boston 1968).

Sandler, G. B.: Improving participant observation: the T-group as an answer. J. appl. behav. Sci. *9:* 31–61 (1973).

Trilling, L.: Sincerity and authenticity (Harvard University Press, Cambridge 1972).

Vansina, L. S.: Aspects psychologiques de la fonction de conseil. Ned. Tijdschr. Psychol. *25:* 3 (1970).

Webb, E. J.; Campbell, D. J.; Schwartz, R. D., and Sechrest, L.: Unobtrusive measures in the social sciences (Rand McNally, Chicago 1966).

Whyte, W. F.: Street corner society; 2nd ed. (University of Chicago Press, Chicago 1955).

Contr. hum. Dev., vol. 2, pp. 113–125 (Karger, Basel 1976)

Chapter 11
Dialectic Man as a Subject in Psychological Research

James C. Mancuso

In the ambience of modern psychology, those who make the claim that man functions as a dialectician must confront the question, 'What is the scientific utility of assuming that a person's behavior reflects his use of a dialectic approach to ordering the universe?' The present chapter offers evidence that empirical psychology has already provided a sound basis for treating a human as if he were a dialectician – that is, as being capable of developing and acting-out an antithesis to every meaning-thesis which he encounters. We begin by distinguishing between two treatments of 'the response', with particular reference to the way in which such behaviors are to be seen recurring over time. On the one hand, we have the view which devolved through British Associationism – a position which holds that a response is first evoked by a stimulus and then stored in memory as a simulacra of the original event to be recalled at some later time. *Neisser* (1967, pp. 281–282) has termed this the *reappearance hypothesis*. In contrast to this hypothesis, one may adopt the *constructive hypothesis*, whereby one assumes 'making a response' depends on a psychological process of locating stimulus events within a system of constructs.

One who accepts the reappearance hypothesis is inclined to regard the flow of responses as being dependent upon the previous contiguous arrangement of stimuli and the reappearing response. The order of the appearance of the response is governed by the order in which the stimulus-response sequence occurred in the previous history of the person. Knowing the history of the person, which allows one to know the nature of the stored idea and the temporal order in which the ideas occurred, one can predict the person's response from knowing which stimulus is associatively linked through temporal contiguity and other mechanisms, to its predictable response. Historically, this approach has been reflected in attempts to specify stimulus-response bond strengths.

Constructivism does not encourage the kinds of direct predictive statements which specify stimulus-response bond strength. Unlike the reappearance hypothesis, which fits closely to mechanistic paradigms, the constructivist hypothesis fits most comfortably into those positions which *Pepper* (1942) classifies as the contextualist paradigms. The core assumptions of the constructivist position are as follows: (1) Every response is a *fresh* construction or reconstruction of the available stimulus situation (*Paivio*, 1974; *Cofer*, 1973). (2) Personal constructions are best represented as an individual's locations of events within an amalgamated and hierarchically arranged series of constructs (*Scott*, 1969; *Mancuso*, 1970). (3) Constructs are the storage units involved in memory function (*Neisser*, 1967). (4) The constructs used by the construing person are *bipolar!* A person cannot incorporate a construct unless it is extracted from his exposure to contrasting stimulus elements. It is impossible *in principle* to form a unipolar construct. (5) Psychological development, with increasing cognitive maturity, accounts for the information-processing or, in our terms, construct-use strategies. Finally, (6) a behaving person develops construction strategies by which he can choose *alternative* locations of events (*Kelly*, 1955; *Bannister and Fransella*, 1971). It is clear that in sum, our assumptions dictate that we treat the subject of our experimental efforts as though he were a *dialectician!* The image of man fostered by classical associationistic theory with its reappearance assumptions simply does not fit what we take to be the object of our study – a human being!

Despite the hegemony of classical associationistic theory in empirical psychology, there are innumerable examples of psychological research literature which reveal that the experimenters began with implicit assumptions that experimental subjects – persons – do in fact employ bipolar constructs. Due to space considerations we will limit our attention to examples drawn from experimental studies relating to assumptions (4) and (5), above. We shall first take up studies of cognitive process, and then move on to certain findings in the area of developmental psychology.

Cognitive Processes and Dialecticism

Psychologists, in their own construing of their discipline, have always used bipolar descriptive categories. We can think of *Jung*'s 'introversion-extraversion' as just one early dialectical dimension which has had great historical impact on the thinking of psychologists. Unlike *Jung*, however, psychologists have missed the opportunity of reflexively ascribing this same construing approach to their subjects. One cannot miss, however, the impetus which *Osgood et al.* (1957) and *Osgood and Richards* (1973) have given to the consideration that people do make *all* their judgments on bipolar scales. In their design of the *semantic* differential, *Osgood* and his group simply took it as the greatest of common sense that people *could* and *would* define stimulus elements in terms of dichotomous, quantitatively graduated, bipolar judgments.

In building the assumptive structure for their hypotheses concerning the semantic basis of the human use of the conjunctions *and* and *but*, *Osgood and Richards* (1973, pp. 385–386) discuss the following two propositions: '*Meaning elements are analysable into simultaneous sets of bi-polar semantic features* (f_{1-n}), *these features being variable in sign and (in the general case)* in *magnitude.* Although linguists and philosophers usually treat semantic features as if they were discretely either-or in nature – and we do this also in our examples, for ease of exposition – it is clear that many features like size, intelligence, and speed vary continuously, as can be seen from the use of quantifiers (John is very tall . . .) *Each semantic feature has a non-arbitrary polarity, one role being cognitively positive* (+) *and the other negative* (–).'

Working from these and other assumptions, *Osgood and Richards* (1973, p. 397) effectively predict the manner in which English-speaking subjects will use the conjunctions *and* and *but*. For example, they predicted that when the paired adjectives used to describe a stimulus event share the same dominant semantic features, the following would hold: 'Preference of *and* over *but* will vary continuously with the similarity of meaning of the paired adjectives. Thus, in the following pairs of adjectives the likelihood of the use of the connective *but* would increase in the order in which the pairs are presented: *ugly* paired with *mean*, *ugly* paired with *cowardly*, *ugly* paired with *brave*, *ugly* paired with *kind*. Clearly, the polarities of these pairs of adjectives are diversely arranged. *Ugly* and *mean* imply aligned polarities, whereas *ugly* and *kind* imply unmatched polarities.

Osgood and Richards (1973) therefore predicted that if a person were to employ the foregoing sets of adjectives to describe Mary or John, there would be a strong likelihood that the conjunction *and* would be used to join the adjectives to like polarities. The adjective *ugly* paired with *kind* (unlike polarities) would be joined by the conjunction *but:* John is *ugly* but *kind*. Subjects join adjectives of like polarities with the conjunction *and*: John is *ugly* and *mean*. These predictions were borne out in the data collections with remarkable precision. Of course, the *Osgood* group does not take these rigorous empirical findings as evidence for the dialectical side to human behavior. As *Kuhn* (1970) so brilliantly argues, a scientist cannot 'find' what he fails to presume as a possibility in his premising 'paradigm' (or, in our terms, *formal construct*). *Osgood*'s paradigm is the traditional one of British Associationism, hence its users fail to assert what we dialecticians dare to see taking place in his data – and that is, convincing evidence for dialectic man as a subject in psychological research!

When *Helson* (1964) conducts and reports his work on adaptation processes, one similarly finds the ubiquitous implicit assumption that persons respond to stimulus events in terms of their location along bipolar judgment scales (see *Avant*, 1971, p. 20, for an eloquent declaration of the value of *Helson*'s theory relative to our thesis). How could one deny that this assumption is being used in explanation of anchoring effects? Investigators predict, and then find support for predictions, that an 'anchor weight' will effect the judgments – in terms of *light-heavy* – that are made on weights located within another range of the *light-heavy* attribute. One must be correct in inferring that the investigator, when he chose the weights that he would use in his study, expected that his subjects would range the weights on their personal, internalized construct *light-heavy*. Similarly, a review of studies employing other judgment scales advises us that the same dialectical principle applies to the use of constructs like *wide-narrow* (*Dinnerstein et al.*, 1968), *few-many* (*Parducci et al.*, 1960), long-time duration, short-time duration (*Behar and Bevan,* 1961), and *long-short* (*Parducci and Marshall,* 1961).

Bevan and Pritchard (1963) obtained results on tonal intensity which support the general data trends found in psychophysical studies which use anchor stimuli. Just as a very light (or very heavy) weight used as an anchor will shift the categorization of other weights in a judged series, so a very 'soft' tone-loudness will shift the categorization of other tones in the series. Further, even though all the subjects whose judgments contributed to the data pool reported an inability to detect the 'softest' anchor tone, their categorizations of the judged stimuli had been affected just as the experimenters had predicted. The anchor had worked to produce a 'contrast effect'. The subject who had been presented with the anchor stimulus judged the other stimulus tones to be louder than did a sample of similar subjects who had not been exposed to an anchor. In comparison with the subjects given the anchor, the control sample (no anchor) consistently judged every tone to be more toward the *soft* end of the *soft-loud* range. It is apparent that contrast involves something 'within the judge', and not 'within the stimulus'. The stimuli are 'contrasted' to something, but one must resist the temptation to believe that these stimuli are contrasted to each other. When we assert the widely accepted dictum 'All judgments are relative', we need to go on to answer the question: 'Relative to what? ' Our position would hold that all judgments are relative to the person's *internalized* bipolar judgment scales.

The work of *Sherif and Hovland* (1961), *Sherif et al.* (1958) and *Hovland et al.* (1957) also reflects progress from the basic assumption that subjects array stimulus events along linear, bipolar scales. Their work is an extension of studies done on the anchoring effect. They have studied the effects of anchors on judgments of social events as stimulus events. They assume the position that events will be 'assimilated' (judged as being a close match) to an anchor stimulus (i. e., the stimulus which is used as a constant comparison stimulus) when the anchor stimulus is close to the series of judged events. Conversely, a series of events will be 'contrasted' to an anchor stimulus when that stimulus lies at a distance from the event series. This formulation assumes that the scale of judgment is *internal* to the subject, and that *close* and *distant* bear a relationship to the subject's internalized scales. This view is highlighted by *Sherif*'s concern with the subject's own categories in the judgment scales which he uses. His position confronts that of scaling technologists like *Thurstone and Chave* (1929), who would construct scales on the assumption that the units within judgment scales are universal to every judge.

The assumptions of *Sherif*'s model consistently have been shown to have utility (*Hovland et al.* 1957; *Sherif et al.*, 1965) in developing understandings of people making social judgments. Subjects who are committed to extreme positions are shown to be willing to judge as being extreme, in the direction opposite to their own, many of those statements which would be judged as moderate by a person whose own position is located at a 'moderate' position on a bipolarized judgment scale. A person strongly committed, for example, to full inclusion of black people into American society, would regard opposition to bussing to be an expression of segregation. In short, a person's own commitments, within his own dialectic systems, effects the quality of the scales he uses to judge the position of other persons.

We cannot overlook the impressive work of *Bieri* and his collaborators; for, among other things, *Bieri* owes a large debt to that influential teacher of many of us, the late Professor *George A. Kelly*, whose constructive alternativism outlook clearly affirms the following dichotomy corollary: 'A person's construction system is composed of a finite number of dichotomous constructs' (*Kelly*, 1955, p. 59). *Bieri et al.*, (1966) have extended the use of the concepts of assimilation and contrast into considerations of the kind of judgments that comprise the psychological workings of the clinical psychologist. They pay homage to the work of *Kelly*, and also acknowledge debts to *Sarbin et al.* (1960) as well as to *Osgood et al.* (1957).

In that *Kelly*'s theory explicitly proposes that man be viewed as a dialectician, every extension of that theory has encouraged adherence to a position that persons locate events within dichotomous cognitive alignments. A survey of the wealth of studies which have developed personal construct theory would take us through the early work of *Bieri* (1955) and *Levy and Dugan* (1956), and through *Bannister*'s (1960, 1962) and *Bannister and Salmon*'s (1966) fascinating work on the people classed as schizophrenic. Other notable studies are those of *Jaspars* (1966), *Landfield* (1971) and *Duck* (1973). *Bannister and Fransella* (1971) give a very readable demonstration of the utility of seeing man to be the dialectician that *Kelly* attempted to make him.

We turn again to a point suggested in the opening statements, i. e., that even a motor act is to be viewed as a process of locating a stimulus within a person's two-dimensional construct matrix. Motor acts are constructions! *Bartlett* (1958) held to this view, though he spoke of schemata rather than of constructions and he was not, as are we, insistent on regarding schemata as localizations within a cognitive space bristling with two-poled dimensions. Motor acts reflect constructions which are involved with the locating of the movable parts of one's body in a spatial ecology. The complexities of motoric constructions revolve about superb cognitive control of the stimuli which can be related to a person's interlocking, space-defining dimensions. Muscle tensions, limb positions, visual cues, antigravity muscle contractions, eye movements, etc., provide the construable stimuli by which a person orients his body and other objects in space.

The movement toward integrating all psychological activity, including motor acts, into one grand class which shall be called construing has been rapidly carried forward by that most influential cognitive theorist, *Piaget*. Repeatedly explicating his propositions that all thought emerges, in epigenetic fashion, from sensorimotor predecessors, *Piaget* has succeeded in attracting the attention of a series of scholars who have aided in developing clearer understandings of how children learn to order events along the spatial dimensions (*White*, 1969; *Laurendeau and Pinard,* 1970; *Denis-Prinzhorn,* 1960). Each of these investigators, adding to the excellent inspiration provided by *Piaget and Inhelder* (1967) and *Piaget et al.* (1964) carries forward the understanding of how children develop the skill of interacting with their spatial ecology. And, we are not surprised to find that the child's mastery of the two-poled coordinate system represents a major achievement in the development of this skill. For example, when a child can impose a fixed, internally represented axis system over a stimulus, regardless of the orientations of the axes within the stimulus array, he can solve innumerable spatial-ordering problems which he could not solve, had he not 'internalized' the coordinate axis system (*Piaget and Inhelder*, 1967, chap. 13). Additionally, one of the best examples of a psychologist explicitly treating his subject as a dialectician is found in *Inhelder and Piaget*'s (1969, chap. 5) empirical analysis of a developing child's approach to the formulation of complementary classes. This fine-tuned analysis presents a substantial framework for understanding how a child goes at the task of arranging events along a bipolar continuum and how he goes about the selection of verbal labels to name the continua he uses. We conclude, therefore, that a wide array of theory and empirical findings in cognitive processes is consistent with the view of subjects as dialecticians. We next turn to a consideration of the role of dialectic in developmental psychology.

The Bipolar Dimension in Developmental Psychology

Space considerations limit the topics to which we can allude, but we would like to begin with a discussion of transposition and *reversal shift* learning as an example of the development of dialecticism in human beings (see our fifth assumption in the introduction, above). A transposition study involves learning a discrimination of two objects that represent 'adjacent' members of a series of objects that can be ranged along what we have elected to call a two-poled construct. A typical situation is as follows: An experimenter prepares a series of six cut-out squares, which he judges to be graded evenly in size – square No. 1 being the smallest, square 2 being enlarged by extending the sides one fourth the length of the sides in squares 1, square 3 being enlarged by adding one fourth to the length of the side of square 2, and so forth, to the sixth square. A child is presented with square 1 and square 2, simultaneously, and is continually informed that he has selected the 'right' square when he picks up square 2. This latter process is repeated until he continuously chooses only square 2.

The subject then is given squares 2 and 3, and he is asked to decide which is the 'right' stimulus within this array. Investigators typically refer to this last exercise as a 'near test'. If the subject chooses square 3, he is said to have chosen on the basis of *transposition*, in that he had learned to respond to the stimulus array be responding to *largeness*, rather than by responding to the stimulus itself. If he regards square 2, in the near test, as the correct stimulus, he is said to have chosen on the basis of *absolute* learning. Observations may be extended. A child trained on squares 1 and 2 is given the opportunity to respond to a presentation of squares 5 and 6. Such a procedure is called a 'far test'. In the far-test procedure one may also speak of transposition, if the subject responds to square number 6, that is, the larger square. One also may speak of the choice of square No. 5 as an absolute response, although the metaphor becomes a bit strained.

If one were to insist on a pure stimulus-response associationistic explanation of learning, he would have a difficult time explaining the transposition effect achieved in the near-test stage of the study, where the subject is asked to choose the 'right' stimulus from the array of squares No. 2 and 3. If reinforcements strengthen the associative bond between the stimulus and the response, then the subject would be acting contrary to expectations when he chooses square No. 3, in the near test. The training, after all, reinforced the associative bond between square 2, as a stimulus, and the choosing of that square, as a response. Why should anyone choose square 3 as the right square after such associationist training?

To begin in a theory which states that all responses represent the locating of stimuli within systems of two-poled constructs allows us to proceed more efficiently toward an explanation of transposition. From this position one can conclude that the subject who responds absolutely, in the near test, responds from the psychologically simple dichotomy, *stimulus present-stimulus absent*. Square 3 is irrelevent to that subject's constructions of the stimulus event presented in the learning task. The subject who renders a transpositional response operates within the psychologically advanced dichotomous construct, *large-*

small. The person's use of the *large-small* construct 'mediates' his learning. The transposing child has previously learned to use a two-poled construct that allows an advanced approach to judgment activities.

Some years ago, *Kuenne* (1946) reported data to support a line of reasoning which attracts the interest of modern advocates of human dialecticism. *Kuenne* hypothesized that children who would be unable to show that they could use the notion *larger than* would be less likely to transpose in the typical transposition experiment. She suggested that one might find a developmental correlate of the propensity to make choices, after training in a typical transposition study, on the basis of *comparatives* rather than on the strength of bonding between the stimulus (the smaller square, for example) and the response (choosing the smaller square). Research in the intervening years has continued to support *Kuenne*'s theory. Older children are more likely to transpose, whereas younger children are more likely to act in terms of absolute reinforcement, thus fulfilling the expectations which would be held by an investigator who thinks in terms of reinforcement of stimulus-response bonding.

Another chain of investigation ties neatly to the general point of *Kuenne*'s thinking. *Kendler* and *Kendler* (1962, 1969 for reviews) have long been the major articulators of the studies of what is known as 'reversal shifting'. The first stage of reversal shift studies involves guiding the subject's selection from among the stimulus array – usually a series of different-sized and different-colored squares. The individual stimuli within the array vary along two judgmental dimensions, i. e., *large-small* and *dark-light.* In the first stage of the study, the investigator might approve only when the subject chooses the *larger* squares. (It would be equally to the point were the initial training to induce the subject to choose the *lighter* squares.) The second training segment begins after the subject reaches a point where he chooses only the stimuli which the investigator wishes him to choose – the *dark* squares, for example. In the second stage of the study, the subject is required to learn to choose other stimuli. In the condition known as the 'reversal shift' condition, the subject must choose those stimuli which fit on the 'opposite' end of the dimension which guided the original choice pattern. If the original training induced the choosing of a *dark* square, the subject in the reversal shift condition must learn to choose a *light* square. Had he been taught to choose the *large* squares, he must now learn to choose the *small* squares, and so forth. Subjects exposed to the second stage, known as the nonreversal shift condition, are required to choose stimuli on the basis of using another judgment scale. If, for example, the subject had first learned to choose *dark* squares, he is required, in the second stage of the study, to learn to choose the *small* squares. He must shift out of the *dark-light* dimension, and he must choose on the basis of the *small-large* continuum, choosing the stimuli located at the *small* end of the dimension.

As one would logically conclude from having studied *Kuenne*'s original thesis, older children solve the reversal shift problem very rapidly, whereas younger children require an extended period of training to solve the reversal shift problem. At the same time, both younger and older children require approximately equivalent levels of training to appropriately solve the shift to another dimension. In other words, the older children learn something during the initial training which can be transferred to the learning during the second part of the training. We are prompted to ask: What psychological process facilitates this transferable learning?

Kendler and Kendler (1962) spell out their explanation in terms of a mediational hypothesis. In short, they would posit mediational processes to explain the transferable benefits of the original learning. During the initial training period, the older subject learns to relate the 'correct' stimulus to the mediational mechanisms which represent *brightness*, for example, and when they are required to shift from choosing dark squares to choosing light squares, these same mediational mechanisms remain applicable. When they shift to yet another dimension, for example, the size-describing dimension, the brightness dimension mediators are no longer applicable. Thus, in the nonreversal shift (better named extradimensional shift) conditions the older subject is at the same relative disadvantage as is the younger subject who has not developed the mediational systems which facilitate the learning of the reversal shift. In short, the system which older children have developed to mediate the responses on the original training is inapplicable in the nonreversal segment, so they are then functioning as would the younger children who have not yet developed the kinds of mediational systems which increase response efficiency during nonreversal learning!

One next asks: What is the nature of the mediating system which facilitates the reversal shift learning? A suitable response to this question would include a phrase which speaks of developed skill in the use of two-poled constructs. Somehow, one can argue, the older child has developed a means of responding to the initial training stimulus array as if he regards the stimuli within his personal system of two-poled constructs. Something happens to the child's cognitive systems – its mediating systems – which allows it to regard the black stimulus as being 'similar' to the white stimulus, while it cannot regard the large stimuli as having a similarity to the black stimuli. The following statement can be related to those assumptions earlier given as the assumptions by which we describe a person as a user of two-poled judgmental dimensions: *The relative advantage which an older child shows in a reversal shift situation derives from the child's having developed information processing approaches which allow him to demarcate clearly the ends of the two-poled dichotomies which he uses in judgmental situations.*

Is there empirical evidence of the development and use of such two-poled dichotomies? The writer would point to the developmental aspects of the data drawn from the Stanford-Binet intelligence scales (*Terman and Merrill*, 1960).

At age 4 years, the average child can successfully complete the following sentences: Brother is a boy, sister is a . . . . . . ; and, The snail is slow, the rabbit is . . . . It will be some time before this average child will be able spontaneously to name the classifying dimensions along which he locates pairs or sets of stimuli. He can be induced, however, by using this technique called 'opposite analogies', to name the end of the continuum opposed to the name already used in the stimulus phrase. The average child aged 4 years can name the *girl* end of the *boy-girl* continuum if given the opposite end – e. g., if the *boy* end is named – and he or she is given an exemplar of the opposing end of the continuum (in this case, a *sister*). The data which have been collected to construct the Stanford-Binet scales, therefore, indicate that something happens to the average 4-year-old child which allows him or her to treat continua as having two clearly demarcated, oppositional ends. An investigator can evoke reponses showing that the child has mastered a strategy for locating stimuli along the kinds of two-poled construct systems which *Osgood and Richards* (1973) so aptly describe.

Considering this bit of evidence and its interpretation, one begins to speculate about the qualitative changes that take place in the mediating systems which, in turn, allow children of approximately kindergarten age to show transfer effects in the standard reversal shift learning investigations. Could it be that the developmental achievement, which produces these transfer effects, involves a development of information-processing strategies which correspond to *the naming of the ends of applicable judgmental dimensions?* Thus, when the child learns to choose *black* squares, he can then more easily learn to choose *white* squares than to choose *large* squares, because his choice of *black* squares automatically signifies the involvement of *white* – the opposite end of the continuum. Before the age of 4 years, the child does not name – and might not recognize the existence of – *two* oppositely valued ends of his dichotomies. Perhaps, he does not name the two oppositely valued ends because he uses dichotomies which have one positive end opposed to a global and amorphous opposing end, and finds no urgency to regard the amorphous end as discrete and namable (see *Inhelder and Piaget*, 1969, chap. 5). At any rate, it appears as if the child who shows transfer in reversal shift problems is also the child who can describe the stimuli within the problem in terms of dimensions which contain two clearly demarcated, labeled ends. There is, indeed, clear evidence for this suggestion in the reversal-shift learning literature (*Koplon*, 1970; *Johnson and White*, 1957; *White and Johnson*, 1969).

Inhelder and Piaget's (1969) treatment of seriation adds immeasurably to an understanding of the processes involved in transposition, and weaves neatly into the comments made above concerning the developing use of bipolar dimensions in human maturation. Seriation is essentially the process of using bipolar dimensions to range stimulus events, a process basic to the human's classifying of experience, and one which is at the core of the mechanistic concept discussed as 'generalization'. To a contextualist, a class is the person's private property, and classes are thought of as constructions that are pragmatically applied to any kind of 'objectively' disparate stimulus events. It is easy to see that these construing processes – this process of class construction and application – are similar to what a literary person might call *metaphor making* (*Turbayne*, 1970). The human being thereby comes to see 'identities among disparities' through construing them within sets of bipolar constructs.

We conclude once again, that a study of the empirical findings in a respected field of psychology, i. e., developmental psychology, is completely in line with a view of the subject as a dialectician. It is the writer's view that a thorough explication of the developmental literature can show us how the dialectical process first appears, how it changes, and how the person employs it throughout life to facilitate his adaptation to the events around him. All we need do is to take on the proper paradigmatic frame of reference in the manner of *Kuhn* (1970) and the rest will fall readily into place.

References

Avant, L. L.: Psychophysics and scaling; in *Appley* Adaptation - level theory (Academic Press, New York 1971).

Bannister, D.: Conceptual structure in thought-disordered schizophrenics. J. ment. Sci. *106:* 1230–1249 (1960).

Bannister, D.: The nature and measurement of schizophrenic thought disorder. J. ment. Sci. *108:* 325–342 (1962).

Bannister, D. and Fransella, F.: Inquiring man (Penguin, Baltimore 1971).

Bannister, D. and Salmon, P.: Schizophrenic thought disorder: specific or diffuse? Br. J. med. Psychol. *39:* 215–219 (1966).

Bartlett, F. E.: Thinking: an experimental and social study (Basic Books, New York 1958).

Behar, I. and Bevan, W.: The perceived duration of auditory and visual intervals. Cross-modal comparison and interaction. Am. J. Psychol. *74:* 17–26 (1961).

Bevan, W. and Pritchard, J. F.: Effect of 'subliminal' tones upon the judgment of loudness. J. exp. Psychol. *66:* 23–29 (1963).

Bieri, J.: Cognitive complexity – simplicity and predictive behavior. J. abnorm. soc. Psychol. *51:* 263–268 (1955).

Bieri, J.; Atkins, A. L.; Briar, S.; Leaman, R. L.; Miller, H., and Tripodi, T.: Clinical and social judgment (Wiley, New York 1966).

Cofer, C. N.: Constructive processes in memory. Am. Sci. *61:* 537–543 (1973).

Denis-Prinzhorn, M.: Perceptions des distances et constance des grandeurs. Etude génétique. Arch. Psychol., Genève *37:* 181–309 (1960).

Dinnerstein, D.; Michel, G. and Byrwa, D.: Inter- and intramural context effects on kinesthetically perceived breadth (unpublished, Rutgers University, New Brunswick 1968).

Duck, S. W.: Personal relationships and personal constructs (Wiley, New York 1973).

Helson, H.: Adaptation level theory (Harper & Row, New York 1964).

Hovland, C. I.; Harvey, O. J., and Sherif, M.: Assimilation and contrast effects in reactions to communication and attitude change. J. abnorm. soc. Psychol. *55:* 244–252 (1957).

Inhelder, B. and Piaget, J.: The early growth of logic in the child (Norton, New York 1969).

Jaspars, J. M. F.: On social perception (Lectura, Leiden 1966).

Johnson, P. J. and White, R. M.: Concept of dimensionality and reversal shift performance in children. J. exp. Child Psychol. *5:* 223–227 (1957).

Kelly, G. A.: The psychology of personal constructs (Norton, New York 1955).

Kendler, H. H. and Kendler, T. S.: Vertical and horizontal processes in problem solving. Psychol. Rev. *69:* 1–16 (1962).

Kendler, H. H. and Kendler, T. S.: Reversal-shift behavior: some basic issues. Psychol. Bull. *72:* 229–232 (1969).

Koplon, D.: Dichotomy in cognition and reversal and non-reversal shifting; unpublished diss., State University of New York, Albany (1970).

Kuenne, M. R.: Experimental investigation of the relation of language to transposition behavior in young children. J. exp. Psychol. *36:* 471–490 (1946).

Kuhn, T. S.: The structure of scientific revolutions; 2nd ed. (University of Chicago Press, Chicago 1970).

Landfield, A. W.: Personal construct systems in psychotherapy (Rand McNally, Chicago 1971).

Laurendeau, M. and Pinard, A.: The development of the concept of space in the child (International Universities Press, New York 1970).

Levy, L. H. and Dugan, R. D.: A factorial study of personal constructs. J. consult. Psycho. *20:* 53–57 (1956).

Mancuso, J. C. (ed.): Readings for a cognitive theory of personality (Holt, Rinehart, & Winston, New York 1970).

Neisser, U.: Cognitive psychology (Appleton Century Crofts, New York 1967; quotations by permission of Prentice Hall, Englewood Cliffs).

Osgood, C. E. and Richards, M. M.: From yang and yin to and or but. Language *49:* 380–412 (1973).

Osgood, C. E.; Suci, G. J. and Tannenbaum, P. H.: The measurement of meaning (University of Illinois Press, Urbana 1957).

Paivio, A.: Language and knowledge of the world. Educ. Researcher *3:* 5–12 (1974).

Parducci, A.; Calfee, R. C., Marshall, L. M., and Davidson, L. P.: Context effects in judgment: adaptation level as a function of mean, midpoint, and median of the stimuli. J. exp. Psychol. *60:* 65–77 (1960).

Parducci, A. and Marshall, L. M.: Context effects in the judgments of length. Am. J. Psychol. *74:* 576–583 (1961).

Pepper, S.: World hypotheses (University of California Press, Berkeley 1942).

Piaget, J. and Inhelder, B.: The child's conception of space (Routledge & Kegan, London 1956; in paperback: Norton, New York 1967).

Piaget, J., Inhelder, B., and Szeminska, A.: The child's conception of geometry (Harper Torchbooks, New York 1964).

Sarbin, T. R.; Taft, R., and Bailey, D. E.: Clinical inference and cognitive theory (Holt, Rinehart, & Winston, New York 1960).

Scott, W. A.: Structure of natural cognitions. J. Personality soc. Psychol. *12:* 261–268 (1969).

Sherif, M. and Hovland, C. I.: Social judgment: assimilation and contrast effects in communication and attitude change (Yale University Press, New Haven 1961).

Sherif, C.; Sherif, M., and Nebergall, R. E.: Attitude and attitude change: the social judgment – involvement approach (Saunders, Philadelphia 1965).

Sherif, M.; Taub, D., and Hovland, C. I.: Assimilation and contrast effects of anchoring stimuli on judgments. J. exp. Psychol. *55:* 150–155 (1958).

Terman, L. M. and Merrill, M. A.: Stanford-Binet intelligence scale (Houghton Mifflin, Boston 1960).

Thurstone, L. L. and Chave, E. J.: The measurement of attitude (University of Chicago Press, Chicago 1929).

Turbayne, C.: The myth of metaphor (University of South Carolina Press, Columbia 1970).

White, B.: The initial coordination of sensorimotor schemas in human infants – Piaget's ideas of the role of experience; in *Elkind and Flavell* Studies in cognitive development (Oxford University Press, New York 1969).

White, R. M. and Johnson, P. J.: Concept of dimensionality and optional shift performance in nursery school children. J. exp. Child Psychol. *6:* 113–119 (1968).

Contr. hum. Dev., vol. 2, pp. 126–150 (Karger, Basel 1976)

Chapter 12
A Summing Up

Joseph F. Rychlak

In Chapter 1, a number of meanings of the dialectic were reviewed for the reader, and it would seem appropriate at this point to look back over the chapters to see if the scheme offered at the outset was relevant to the actual dialectical formulations employed in the intervening chapters. We should also look into some of the potential dangers in use of dialectical constructions, and consider some of the reasons for rejecting the dialectic which are commonly heard. It should be noted that the interpretations and arguments of this chapter are solely those of the writer, and that they do not necessarily reflect the collective views of the contributors. As *Sardello* noted in Chapter 3, dialecticians are likely to have their own views on things which makes them appear contentious. This is no less true when we consider the essentials of the dialectical metaconstruct itself. We begin, then, by looking at the interpretations of dialectic actually employed by the contributors to this volume.

Dialectical Formulations of the Contributors

Since the editor asked only that the contributors provide the reader with a clear picture of how he or she viewed the dialectic vis-à-vis the particular topic under presentation, there was no effort to prearrange usages. Chapter 1 was written independently of and before the rest of the chapters, and therefore its categorizations were not directly influential on the writings of the contributors. In light of this, can we see these categories in the various topics discussed in the volume? We will now attempt an interpretative overview of the uses of dialectic to be seen in the chapters of this volume, with parenthetical references to the five meanings of dialectic discussed in Chapter 1 (i. e., World Principle, Valid Organon, Invalid Organon, Transcendence, and Many in One or vice versa).

Sardello's conception of the dialectic is individualized, an intrapersonal focus on the aesthetic experience or the humorous delight taken in the many-faceted aspects of life (many in one). We see a Socratic emphasis in the dialogue which the aestheticist generates between himself and the art object. The greater the cultivation of this dialogue, the richer and more diverse is the aesthetic experience (valid Organon). Similarly, in humor there is a dialogical mode of experience in which, although not always generated by dialogue, things are found to be more involved and surprising than they were at first (transcendence). In the aesthetic experience the person may generate these alternatives by relating to the art object and seeing it many ways, take delight in the totality of the different – even contradictory – meanings to be generated there. In humor, a person seems more taken by surprise, delighted in the unexpected turn of events. Of course, in humor based on setting oneself above others there can be an element of intended superiority (as, in humor which denigrates a minority group). But much of the effect of generating laughter, as *Sardello* demonstrates, is brought forth by the incongruity of a sudden insight in which things are what they are not. And, of course, the aspect of humor which *Sardello* describes as a conversation initiated with the opposite side of our natures is clearly in the vein of a Socratic dialectic.

This internal dialogue is what *Rychlak* also finds in Freudian psychoanalysis. The one person becomes three (id, ego, super-ego as many in one), and a possibility for alternatives 'initiated from within' exists (as a form of transcendence), in which conflict and compromise are often generated. Symptomatology as character traits are taken as syntheses of contradictory intentions (wishes), so that there is probably more of a need for resolving the contradictions in this subjective dialectic than *Sardello* would say is required in the aesthetic or humorous situation. The Freudian dialectical conception is used 'dynamically' to account for how a person's motivations take seed and manifest themselves 'both at once' (i. e., a synthesis). Yet in another sense it is probably true that Freudian compromises are not true syntheses because the two sides are never really made 'one'. *Freud*'s genius lay in teasing out the two sides to the compromise, and, in this exposure obviating the need for a more permanent joining of the conflicting intentionalities.

Datan's presentation moves the dialectic outward, into the realm of the interpersonal. One might argue that male versus female is a kind of physically-based inevitability in the human circumstance (world principle), but *Datan*'s treatment emphasizes that there is an implicit, reciprocal definition between the sexes which is not itself fixed to biology or even to culture *per se*. One side defines the other, and however these two patterns of sexual behavior come to be manifested, the essential point is that they do share the meaning of their opposite member (one in many). Indeed, we are all divided identities – women and men – desirous of uniqueness yet seeking a temporary synthesis in sexual union. The role of the offspring and the family unit then enters to fix life-styles for a period, but in the life cycle we also witness a convergence and reversal of roles over time (transcending familiar patterns, and taking up the opposite).

Hogan's description of the dialectic encompassed the individual conception which *Sardello* and *Rychlak* had employed, stressing the thought form used by a social scientist who construes events from the perspective of organicism, and hence arrives at a different conceptualization than does the more conventional, demonstrative scientist (valid organon). There is, however, the beginning here in Chapter 6 of the significant idea that each successive hypothesis passing through dialectical machinations (thesis, antithesis, synthesis) forms into a progressively more satisfactory statement of things. This interpretation of dialectic is Hegelian (world principle), although *Hogan* is not employing it in the sense of a supra-individual progression in events. He, as *Kierkegaard* had done, draws from the Hegelian conception as a kind of analogy to the individual (*Kierkegaard*'s subjective dialectic). But the concept of a *developmental* progression or advance is then made possible, for it is predicated on the view that what eventuates over dialectical resolutions is the 'best' of what had gone before as contradictory bipolarities. Far from heralding the dissolution of progression, discontinuity and conflict are the well-spring of positive advance.

A similar developmental conception is held to by *Riegel*, who emphasizes the Hegelian (world principle) theme that contradiction is basic to all motion and vitality. The focus of *Riegel*'s chapter is on cognitive development *per se* (valid organon). In opposition to *Piaget*, *Riegel* suggests that individual development in thought is *not* away from contradiction and denial toward the untrammeled unidirectionality and certainty of abstract thinking. He points to the unappreciated role of cultural-historical conditions, conditions which also enter in to determine the quality of developmental stages in thought. Moreover, *Riegel* admonishes that while stages occur in thought, we must not confuse such structures with the (dialectical) process. In transforming contradictory experience into stable structures we witness the products of thinking, but not thinking *per se* (a variant form of the one-and-many thesis).

Kuo's chapter teaches us that the writing style of the *I Ching* (valid organon) reflecting the traditional *yin-yang* principle of Chinese thought (world principle) prepared the Eastern intellect for an easy acceptance of the Hegelian-Marxian formulations of modern Communism (world principle). *Kuo* suggests that unlike Westernized views of the dialectic in social forces, where the contradiction and opposition of this process are held to eventuate in a social explosion of class warfare, the Chinese are more ready to see in this dialectical confrontation a balancing eventuality short of such dramatic eruptions (one and many). Chinese thinkers have been seen as passive and even weak because of their willingness to accept inconsistency and not demanding thereby a settlement of the question into a synthesis, much less a victory of one side over the other. The unique feature of Eastern thought has always been that it could see the harmony in disharmony. It is probably at least in part for this reason that *Mao* could so readily find a continuing role for the dialectic in the self- and group-criticism practices of the Chinese peoples following the Revolution.

Kvale performs a kind of dialectical twist on the critic of dialectic, the one who is likely to claim that 'facts speak for themselves' and hence any concept which embraces dualities and contradictions in the factual is by definition sophistical and invalid (the invalid organon contention). *Kvale*'s argument hinges upon the view of man as dialectically facing alternatives in his description of behavior, and hence, having to affirm 'this' or 'that' interpretation of events rather than simply finding his facts as pebbles on a beach (many and one). Having some modicum of arbitrariness in how he may see things, the role of *values* in what he does claim to see enters in as a selective precedent factor. Only someone with a naively demonstrative view of things can sincerely believe that facts come packaged in value-free boxes. *Kvale*'s stress on praxis flows directly from this assumption that facts are always tools in social relations, and, of course, can therefore align themselves with class attitudes. The argument draws from Hegelian-Marxian themes (world principle) at this point, since the assumption is made – in contrast to the thesis of *Kuo* concerning Oriental contradictions – that a contest is being worked out in historical events.

The theme of qualitative changes (structures, etc.) taking place over the course of time in a positively developing direction would have been termed by *Kierkegaard* the movements (leaps) across 'stadia'. *Kierkegaard*'s view of change is quite in contrast to the efficient-cause conceptions of change so prevalent in psychology today. *Hogan*'s talk of definable endpoints to dialectical development, *Riegel*'s distinction between thought structures and the process of thinking, and *Kvale*'s emphasis on the qualitative changes brought about through the development of internal contradictions are all directly traceable to the Kierkegaardian conception of change, as well as to the Hegelian view on which it was based. Newtonian science accepted the demonstrative world view of unidirectional, equal-staged changes in events, but there is good reason to see in modern physics a more dialectical outlook as in *Bohr*'s discontinuous world of nature where electrons no longer move about in just any orbit encircling the atomic nucleus. *Feuer* (1974, p. 138) has made the interesting case that *Bohr's* theoretical rationale emanated from the Kierkegaardian inspiration of his teacher, *Harφld Hoffding.* If so, it must be pointed out that ultimately this inspiration and influence emanated from dialectical conceptualization *per se,* something which has a history in the thought of mankind far transcending any one person or even epoch in lived time.

The Newtonian conception of unidirectionality and linearity hence a mathematized form of change takes us directly into *Lourenço*'s efforts to delineate the essentials of a qualitative methodology. This amounts to, if not a direct opposition, then at least an alternative research strategy to the classical quantitative methods of science. Qualitative differences are differences in kind, idiographically unique circumstances similar to the Kierkegaardian and Hegelian stages or stadia in the unfolding of some (historical or individual-life) theme. *Lourenço* is proceeding on the assumption that human experience is not additive. One cannot even predict the course of these changes based on the assumption of a unidirectional, efficiently caused thrust in events from out of the past. When such abrupt, qualitative shifts occur, the typical quantitative psychologist assumes that his parameter has shifted and lets it go at that. His method is therefore inevitably incomplete, nondefinitive, and even *post hoc* – catching the frozen points without being able to account for the process of change (as per *Riegel*'s arguments above). Quantitative methods require that something go before them, some paradigm, some approach to what they will call 'data' and 'variables' when they get around to putting such 'facts' (see *Kvale*) to test. Qualitative methodology seeks to capture the total process, and, in doing so, invariably comes upon dialectical themes in the actual behavior of people – experimenter as well as subject.

Lourenço thus entered the 'data source', and, looking at the process under study from the same perspective as the subjects of her study, attempted to delineate what was actually taking place in this more fluid sense of change through conflict and negotiation (valid organon). She used a Socratic-Platonic interpretation of the dialectic to capture this process and also to retain a certain marginality by turning back on herself as a person to test her influence on and reactions to the data being delineated (transcendence). *Lourenço* placed an emphasis on the dialectic which may be thought of as distinctive from all other views to this point, in that she recognized that the dialectic did not solve problems for all time. The dialectic seemed to enter into both problem solution and problem generation in human relations. This may be a variant of *Sardello*'s assessment of the dialectical intelligence as contentious or problem-generating, but there is at least the suggestion in addition that dialectic *per se* cannot be counted on to close every issue that it opens up! Even so, *Lourenço* did accept the developmental thesis we have seen emerge in the chapters by *Hogan*, *Riegel* and *Kvale* – i. e., of an improvement over the course of dialectical progression because it necessarily encompasses all that has gone before it. We might say that when a synthesis *is* closed we note a progression, but that it does not follow that all such antithetical contradictions do in fact get synthesized into a new totality.

In taking up questions of validity and reliability, *Lourenço* also reflected her sensitivity to the frequent charges made by demonstrative thinkers to the effect that dialectical formulations, since they allow so many alternatives in the accrual of knowledge, are nonscientific or at least sub-professional (invalid organon). It is certainly true that the dialectician often takes an interest in and accepts as valid information what is called 'error variance' by the quantitative methodologist. To the demonstrative intellect, something either *is* or *is not* (law of contradiction). Hence, when a series of measurements are accumulated and put into a frequency dispersion, it is assumed that only *one* of the points on the dimension of distribution touches – or, comes closest to touching – upon a substrate reality (i. e., the population parameter). A dialectician is more likely to see such averages as the mean and median as purely fictional inventions, useful but not necessarily any more 'true' than the variance in measurement to be seen dispersing around the central tendency of an array of measurements. And what are we to do if we find by entering the frequency distribution in the manner of *Lourenço*'s qualitative method that some of the measures which departed from the central tendency measure were not simply 'chance', but were based on intentional strategies of the human beings under study? At this point, the quantitative methodologist can do nothing but shrug his shoulders and find a different, more cooperative sampling of data on which to base his assessments of what 'is' without troubling himself to account for what 'is not'.

This third-person or *extraspective* outlook of quantitative methodology, encouraging a nomothetic form of science is what qualitative methodology seeks to counterbalance (see *Rychlak*, 1968, pp. 27–34). Dialecticians (not all, but most!) are more ready to take a first-person or *introspective* perspective in their construction of the scientific task, to see how things are progressing from the slant of the data (i. e., human beings) under observation. This makes no sense in natural science, where often inanimate events are under description, but an introspective perspective is all-important to the social sciences. Dialectical logic is sensitive to values (*Kvale*) because at heart this is a logic of the implications in events. The dialectician invariably sees events progressing 'from this point onward', utilizing the past as the source of alternative premises about what shall take place in the henceforth. Given 'this' view of the past, 'such and thus' will follow. Given 'that' view of the past, 'thus and such' will follow. Which view of the past is the correct one? At this point, dialecticians may well disagree, for this is a question concerning the content of the dialectical progression. We are not interested in the present volume in the specific contents of any *one* theory, although obviously our contributors felt that their particular realm of interest was important to them in framing their chapters (as well as to certain of their readers). But what we are striving for in the present volume is an understanding of the style of dialectics *per se.* And this style has been seen to draw us ever to the more introspective slant of things, looking where possible at the world through the eyes of our experimental subjects.

When we do so, *Mancuso* draws our attention to the fact that they too reason dialectically, i. e., through bipolarities termed 'constructs' which can be framed from any of a number of perspectives (many and one) and which amount to a predicate assumption regarding the world of experience (both valid and invalid organon). We lose the global, supraindividual treatment here of some of the intervening chapters and return to the more person-centered conception of the dialectic with which the book had begun. We also lose the dialectical developmental emphasis, for, although *Mancuso* speaks of the capacity for dialectical reasoning to function more or less in development, he does not actually have a theory which suggests that the dialectic is *in* development or is the contradictory cause of development. Children are shown to develop information-processing strategies which permit them to demarcate more clearly the ends of two-poled, cognitive dichotomies in maturation. But the maturation *per se* is left unanalyzed and to this extent might be thought of in the traditional unipolar, unindirectional and linear sense of the demonstrative reasoner. Even so, the basic insight on which *Mancuso* builds his case is a dialectical one. It stresses the bipolarity in meanings, and how these multifaceted meanings can permit the subject of an experiment to behave in the fashion in which he is observed behaving.

This does not mean that *Mancuso* would necessarily disagree with a more clearly dialectical conception of development as advocated by *Riegel* or *Hogan*, of course; nor does it mean that *Mancuso*'s analysis is irrelevant to the latter viewpoints. *Mancuso*'s chapter is especially important to the total argument of the present volume, for it demonstrates convincingly that even on the demonstrative reasoner's most sacrosanct grounds of 'the laboratory', dialectical formulations meet the challenge of accounting for the findings actually observed. One is not actually predicting the direction of a dialectical progression in these laboratory findings, but without a dialectical construction of the 'data' we do not obtain the same degree of understanding of the cognitive processes involved. *Mancuso*'s chapter concretizes *Kvale*'s arguments by showing how the preferred paradigm of lab-psychologists predetermine the 'facts' they supposedly find at play before their 'unbiased' eyes. It also shows that one need not employ *Lourenço*'s qualitative methodology, as a dialectician. Qualitative methodology may be essential in certain types of studies, but even after one has delineated the variables of importance and nailed down a procedure suitable to the laboratory, relying upon dialectical conceptualizations in a quantitative methodological context is also fruitful and even necessary.

Cautions in the Use of Dialectical Formulations

The writer feels that there are certain cautions to be cited in the use of dialectical formulations. The most general caution is that a theorist be absolutely certain that he really has a dialectic in mind when he is using this term (this was also discussed in Chapter 1). Some theorists use the term loosely as a synonym for difference, or, diametric opposite. If one does not begin with some basic idea to the effect that a given (thesis) either immediately defines or at least distinctly implies its opposite (antithesis), then one is not basing his theoretical development on a true dialectic, even though it may be that an analogy is being drawn to a dialectical construct. For example, when we say that white is the opposite of black, or that oil and water are opposites we draw such an analogy. Furthermore, it should be possible in principle for a demonstrative reasoner to speak of opposition in events without thereby having to admit to being dialectical.

Demonstrative views of opposition or difference are not based on a bipolarity in meaning, but rather on a unipolarity. Something is said to be different from something else if some quality in question – a *single* quality – is unequally distributed across the two cases in point. Thus, the demonstrative reasoner might say that being wet from rain is opposite to being dry, thinking now in terms of the quality of moisture as unevenly distributed across the two circumstances. Or, two things might be said to be diametrically opposite which are at different ends of some designated *single* dimension – as a kind of 'apposed' notion. For example, if a linear scale has units running from 0 to 100, the demonstrative reasoner might say that a value of 0 is diametrically opposite to 100. Yet the score of 0 does not *by definition* imply this opposite score of 100. Once again, the lesson for a dialectician is to examine his conception carefully in light of what there is about it to make it truly reflective of the dialectic.

Another caution which the writer would advance concerns the belief expressed by several of our contributors to the effect that because it always subsumes or takes account of what has gone before, a dialectical progression must always be an improvement over what had transpired earlier. Though this may be true in certain instances, it is hardly a tenet to be embraced as a necessary feature of the dialectic. We are reminded here of *Aristotle*'s original dissatisfaction with dialectic as organon (see Chapter 1, invalid organon). His point was that two participants in a Socratic dialogue did not necessarily begin their conversational course in truth, hence they could not necessarily hope to improve on this and end in truth. We might add that even if this series had been initiated in truth, thanks to the multiplicity in dialectical reasoning it is conceivable that the path of development could have taken a false turn at some point and now 'all that had gone before' could be directing events in anything but a positive direction. Furthermore, as we noted above in discussing *Kvale*'s paper, the past is always subject to reinterpretation, so that even when earlier problems have been solved successfully, there is no assurance that one's review of what has already transpired will necessarily add up to a sound assumption today concerning the henceforth.

In a physical sphere of explantion, as in the development of skills based upon the dialectic of maturation and a coordinate experience of having lived for 'so long', the progressive features of dialectical development might be shown to be true, particularly over certain periods of the life span. But in other applications of the dialectic this assumption seems highly dubious. Take both Hegel's and Marx's employment of the dialectic, which rested on the assumption of positive movement over time; both men *ended* their dialectic in the supposed 'best' circumstance of an enlightened Prussian monarchy and a classless state, respectively. Ironically, two of the greatest dialecticians of history thus stopped employing the construct when it suited their theoretical purposes to do so (a point mentioned in Chapters 1 and 8). Surely, as the present volume demonstrates, the sagacious dialectician would not only be likely to contest the ending of dialectic in the march of civilization, but he would have a few alternative points to make concerning what is 'best' in this world of shifting realities.

Although *Kvale* would probably disagree, this is not simply a political statement. It is a recognition at the level of theory that dialectics will simply never end, and that one can – through valuations of circumstances – always call into question what 'is' by way of 'what is not'. Hence, to suggest that one view is bourgeois and a second proletarian, or, one revolutionary and a second counter-revolutionary is simply to put historical meat on the dialectical frame. This frame can be seen working from either perspective, and to the advantage of either side. Which point of view will prevail is hardly dictated by the frame, and belief in a dispersion of this conflictual frame in time is an optimistic act of faith which neither history nor knowledge of dialectic would seem to support. Indeed, if the human animal is dialectical by nature, then it seems unlikely that such a frame could drop from view – either at the sociocultural or individual level of behavioral description. To assume that the 'best' will eventuate thanks to successive dialectical resolutions of past contradictions is to take an uncharacteristic, unidirectional attitude toward the march of events. This is why the writer finds it sound to agree with *Lourenço* that, in the final analysis, the dialectic is not suited to ending problems as absolutely solved. And, we may be certain that once we can predict the course of dialectic, we are no longer speaking as dialecticians but as demonstrative reasoners who have caught the tide of a unidirectionality in events.

This question also shades into the third caution we have, and that is: avoid taking a doctrinaire view of dialectics. As the present volume surely establishes, there is no formula of 'thesis-antithesis-synthesis' which must be met before we consider a theorist to be a dialectician. If we are going to insist that there must be a synthesis in every dialectical formulation, then we not only begin intruding with demonstrative, unidirectional claims but we overlook the fact that two or more lines of argument can be carried on as parallels at the *same* time. Creative individuals in all walks of life are constantly sensitive to such dual implications in events. The meaning of a circumstance which seems to shift from moment to moment may appear unreliable to the demonstrative reasoner, but to a dialectician who assumes the proper perspective the reversals and involutions in events (the 'error variance', see above) are not without their logic. Too many people think that dialectic means the Hegelian formula of 'thesis-antithesis-synthesis' and nothing else. We naturally hope that the present volume has served to dispel this erroneous notion.

Rejection of Dialectic Based on Its Misunderstood Role in Science

The writer has found that it is almost a certainty following his speaking on the topic of dialectic that a critic arises in the audience to attack the construct on the grounds of its unscientific nature. The criticism takes three general forms. The first has to do with the use of terms and the loss of universal precision to be seen in dialectical definitions: 'How can we be scientific based on the view that there is an opposite to everything? What's the opposite of green? ' It must then be pointed out that we do not propose an either/or choice need be made between dialectical and demonstrative conceptualizations in *every* case. Only when the dialectical formulation naturally meets the material to be described should it be used. *Of course*, there is no opposite to every conceptualization excepting only in that analogical sense of saying 'green exists' implies 'no green exists'. In this case, existence is the meaning having a properly dialectical frame which is then analogically extended to the affirmation 'green'. But surely there can be referential designations which are *not* oppositional. The nouns of our language are in large measure without opposites, reflecting as they do a summary of qualities signifying a uniformity as a 'thing'.

But when we look at the modifying qualities of things, we find there a host of dialectical meanings. Colors are nondialectical designations, but other essentially psychological descriptive qualities, which locate an item in space, relate it to some personal impression, or evaluate it preferentially are almost always dialectical ascriptions. Left-right, aggressive-passive, liked-disliked, etc., are the touchpoints of human subjective awareness and objective reality. *Mancuso*'s review (Chapter 11) made it unquestionably clear that insofar as psychological scientists have made sense of their area, they have fallen back on such bipolar descriptions – as do *all* people. Hence, the fact that we can point to unipolar designations does not in itself demolish the dialectic as a useful and necessary formulation of scientific observations.

The second objection from a scientific perspective takes the form: 'You contend that the course of dialectic cannot be predicted. How then are we to have a science of behavior if it does not predict behavior? ' This question rests on the fact that, in order to validate one's scientific theory, it is necessary to 'control and predict' in the act of validation (*Rychlak*, 1968, p. 77). We apply controls to variables, holding some constant, and manipulating the independent variables in order to observe their effects on dependent variables – effects which have themselves been predicted to occur beforehand. The erroneous implication taken from this is that science is dedicated to the literal prediction of events.

This demonstrative line of thought would therefore find a conception of nonpredictability to be contrary to science on the face of things.

Of course, whether or not human behavior is predictable or unpredictable is no measure of the legitimacy of a science of behavior *per se*. This line of criticism conveniently overlooks the fact that unpredictability is part and parcel of every experiment conducted in psychology. If we were to draw conclusions from the amount of variance accounted for in most experiments on human beings, surely a balanced view would be that much and usually most of behavior is *un*predictable. And when we look at experiments in which the dialectical reasoning capacities of a human subject may be thought to take place – i. e., thinking, creativity, verbal conditioning, etc. – we find evidence that what we *do* learn through experimentation is contingent upon the subject's ability to grasp and conform to the experimental instructions we give him. The vast contribution which a subject's premises, beliefs, or awareness of the experimental procedures play in his actual performance reflected in our 'data' cannot be doubted (*Dulany*, 1962; *Orne*, 1962; *Rosenthal*, 1966). And when we approach the experimental situation taking *both* the experimenter's and the subjects' grasp of these circumstances into consideration, we learn that subjects can and do cooperate or fail to cooperate with the experimenter's expectations *at will* (*Page*, 1972).

If this is true, then from what source in the experimental design does the so-called predictability take root? Is it completely discernible 'in' the extraspectively observed events, or, must we first get over into the heads of our subjects in the manner of *Lourenço* and learn what *they* construe as taking place, and whether *they* want to conform to experimental expectations or not? And if the vaunted predictability of our experiments stems from the latter factors, then clearly we are capitalizing on a major form of 'unknown' in our actuarial rule. Since the experimenter cannot predict the extent of this cooperation for any subject, but must settle for the cooperation he does receive, is it not simple honesty to admit that subjects who refuse to be studied in the first place, or, when studied, who purposely confound the experimental procedure, are not simply part of an unintentional error variance, but are *dialectically* opting for the unpredictiveness observed? Surely we are now mature enough in social science to acknowledge this aspect of our scientific work. This recognition does not detract from the general logic of science. The dialectic helps us to understand our rigorous procedures in ways that demonstrative strategies have no appreciation for. Far from detracting from science, dialectic strengthens it.

Another misunderstanding in the criticism relying on the lack of predictability in dialectical progressions is that they erroneously assume that a scientist is supposed *literally* to be predicting behavior. There can be no argument with the fact that, in doing an experiment, all psychologists 'control and predict' in an attempt to validate their hypotheses. But, whether or not science is next called on to apply such knowledge *as science* is a question much in dispute. The distinction between basic and applied science stems from precisely this question of whether or not psychologists are supposed to spend their lives as behavioral actuarians. This is what 'predicting behavior' would come down to, for as *Atkinson* (1974, p. 408) pointed out, even when a substantial correlation is found between personality variables of various sorts, this describes 'the modal personality of a particular society at a particular time in history'. Hence, to formulate one's role as a literal 'predictor of behavior' rather than as an 'explainer of behavioral principles' places one in the role of a sociohistorical actuarian, seeking ever newer, more up-to-date samplings from the universe parameter. *Cronbach* (1975, pp. 125–126) seemed to favor such a role for the psychologist, although he acknowledges that there are problems in this activity:

> The forecast (prediction) of Y from A, B, and C will be valid enough, if conditions D, E, F, etc., are held constant in establishing and in applying the law. It will be actuarially valid, valid on the average, if it was established in a representative sample from a universe of situations, as long as the universe remains constant. When the universe changes, we have to go beyond our actuarial rule. As Meehl . . . has said, when we step outside the range of our experience, we have to use our heads.

The dialectician would add that when universes change and we then 'use our head' to detect what the demonstrative actuarial rule itself cannot detect, the reasoning strategy by which this new understanding will be accomplished will be fundamentally dialectical! In fact, any time we set about delineating a universe on which to base our parametric statistic, the same issues arise as in *Kvale*'s discussion of the factual in knowledge (Chapter 9). The initial delineation of a universe as its understanding when changes arise concerning what it relates to are 'figured out' by an intellect which is not quasi-mathematical and cybernetic, but rather thoroughly at ease with inconsistency, two lines of contradictory argument at once, being and non-being, and so forth. *Only* such an intellect would have a 'head' to use once the facts slip past it. Hence it is naive to say that dialectic is nonscientific because it is not *in principle* something which can be predicted. We might as well say that statistical analysis is not scientific, because the universes which it tests change mysteriously and without notice, hence there is a constant breakdown in predictability.

The final criticism we are likely to hear in the form of dialectic's unscientific quality runs as follows: 'How can we be certain that a scientist who accepts dialectic won't try to use it to explain his data as he sees fit, turning empirical findings against his hypothesis into findings for his hypothesis? ' The most direct rebuttal here is to ask whether the questioner honestly believes that such sophistry is not *already* being carried on in the social sciences? *Post hoc* theoretical predictions abound in psychology. And even if they did not, a concern of this sort is ironical since it suggests that dialectical twists in behavior *do* take place, but that we should avoid admitting to them by denying that man has this capacity in the first instance. However, there is a deeper implication in this question, concerning which the writer must again reiterate his plea for a 'personal view'. That is, so long as we distinguish clearly between what is our *theory* and what is our *method* of proving this theory true or false – however lightly we carry these conceptions of truth and falsity – there should be no problem (*Rychlak,* 1975).

Due to their suppleness and reversiblility, dialectical conceptions strike the writer as better suited to the realm of theoretical constructions. Dialectical reasoning is also important to what is often called theoretical proof, or, the plausibilities of common sense which the writer has termed procedural evidence (*Rychlak*, 1968, p. 75). But when it comes to the strictures of scientific methodology, there is no substitute for demonstrative reasoning, which eventuates in validating evidence (i. e., control and prediction to a criterion, as per our discussion above). This is not to deny a role for *Lourenço*'s qualitative methodology, in which the dialectic played such a prominent role (Chapter 10). It is simply to observe that, after qualitative methods have delineated the dimensions along which follow-up work can take place, the more conventional demonstrative logic of quantitative methods can then be introduced. It is no more sensible to ignore quantitative methods entirely than it is to ignore qualitative methods entirely in the work of science.

And so it is that, even if *Lourenço* had somehow twisted findings in an (even unconscious) attempt to present them according to her personal biases, the succession of work done on the area of social conflict, both qualitatively by others and, in time, by extensions into the more well-controlled laboratories, could be counted on to rectify the situation. We may never be able to take an entire television station into the laboratory, but, following the lead of participant-observers like *Lourenço*, we should be able to delineate bits and pieces of our theories about social conflict which have direct relevance to the actual field of television. Psychologists like to speak of the generalizability of findings. They speak as if it is the research data actually found which is supposed to extend somehow by way of magically existing 'laws' from one research collection to another, and another, eventually reaching the 'outside the laboratory' realm of everyday observation, fixed into one grand scheme of 'natural lawfulness'. This is nothing but a *theory* which has been analogized from the methodological context. What always generalizes is not one's research findings (method), but one's theoretical statements about these findings. There are no such things as 'generalizing laws'! Laws are simply observed findings in a methodological context. They rely initially on theories which frame the experiments conducted – or, as *Kuhn* (1970) calls them, *paradigms.* Laws are only laws because our precedent paradigms framed an area of study, enabling us to define our experimental variables, and, in the subsequent process of control and prediction, to demonstrate some kind of relationship between them – i. e., a 'law'! To believe in laws as somehow existing in reality is to confound methodological with theoretical activities of science. It is the *sine qua non* in hypostatization, now widely rampant in all of the 'best' circles of rigorous psychology.

The Possibility of a Humanistic Psychology

As stated in its opening pages, this volume was conceptualized from the outset by the writer as a kind of 'opening shot' in the battle against complete subjugation of psychology to demonstrative, mechanistic images of the person. The term humanism today is badly mangled by all sorts of unhappy connotations, yet we can think of no better term to oppose to mechanism and, therefore, we insist on using it. There is a tendency to confound the meanings of humanism and humanitarianism. Because telic philosophies and theologies have been associated in the history of thought with conceptions of freedom, free-will, and so forth, an unfortunate development we see taking place in the present is to presume that a humanist *must* argue for the more uplifting, quasi-religious side to human behavior. Some psychologists who might honestly want to give humanistic theory serious consideration in their work are dissuaded from doing so because of the goody-goody connotation that humanism has taken on.

Humanism has been identified with encounter groups, and social reform of various types, and even with groups of 'fulfilled' psychologists, dancing around a park bench during the breaks at their professional meetings. It therefore appears that a related admonition of the humanistic approach is to 'see thy brother human being as worthy of respect and help' or some such. Desirable as this might be for a general approach to human relations, such ethical pronouncements are unquestionably harmful to an objective assessment of the data we must think about collecting, manufacture, and then examine as impartially as possible in the rigorous context of empirical research. Not understanding that man's *theoretical* dehumanization arises due to the demonstrative predilection of most psychologists now in positions of political influence in professional and academic circles, the humanist vainly tries to force his tough-minded counterpart to present mankind in a more humanistic fashion. This is a misguided effort. Better to follow *Jung*'s (1961, p. 79) insight that human beings are no more elevated than they are submerged.

If a psychologist is really theorizing in order to raise man's dignity, as *Rogers* (1961) has seemed to do, or, if he is pitching his psychology at an application to human welfare, as *Skinner* (1971) has seemed to do, then *both* such theorists might be said to be *humanitarian* in outlook. The former is a humanistic humanitarian and the latter, a mechanistic humanitarian. There is no reason why all humanists have to be humanitarians. As the writer has argued elsewhere (*Rychlak*, 1975), a theorist's position on this humanistic-mechanistic dimension is not to be discerned from his personal hopes for mankind, nor through his wish that man's dignity be elevated through thinking good thoughts. A theorist's position is to be determined solely on the basis of his employment of certain theoretical devices.

Mechanists put their trust in exclusive reliance on the nontelic, demonstrative conceptions of natural science. Humanists *can* take an alternative approach to science by employing the dialectic in some fashion. As we hope this volume has amply demonstrated, the dialectic provides us with a rationale for theoretical descriptive accounts which show men and women to be telic animals (Chapter 4), conceptually active throughout their development on earth (Chapter 7), with evaluative proclivities making them responsive to the moral side of their behavior (Chapter 6), open to the aesthetic and the humorous in existence (Chapters 2 and 3), seeking identity and heterosexual union with others (Chapter 5), and in a way which is not culture-bound (Chapter 8). It seems fair to say that it is precisely these sort of things which one refers to in the designation 'human being'. There is nothing in science and the knowledge accrued thereby to negate this view of behavior (Chapters 9–12). It is the sincere hope of the editor and other contributors to this volume that the reader can see the legitimacy of this claim, and that we might witness a growing number of people in the social sciences who will turn their interests to an even more active elaboration of the dialectic in years to come.

References

Atkinson, J. W.: Motivational determinants of intellective performance and cumulative achievement; in *Atkinson and Raynor* Motivation and achievement (Winston, Washington 1974).

Cronbach, L. J.: Beyond the two disciplines of scientific psychology. Am. Psychol. *30:* 116–127 (1975).

Dulany, D. E.: The place of hypotheses and intentions: an analysis of verbal control in verbal conditioning; in *Eriksen* Behavior and awareness: a symposium of research and interpretation, p. 102–129 (Duke University Press, Durham 1962).

Feuer, L. S.: Einstein and the generations of science (Basic Books, New York 1974).

Jung, C. G.: The development of personality; in *Read, Fordham and Adler* The collected works of C. G. Jung, vol. 17. Bollingen Series XX.17 (Pantheon Books, New York 1961).

Kuhn, T. S.: The structure of scientific revolutions; 2nd. ed. (The University of Chicago Press, Chicago 1970).

Orne, M. T.: On the social psychology of the psychological experiment: with particular reference to demand characteristics and their implications. Am. Psychol. *17:* 776–783 (1962).

Page, M. M.: Demand characteristics and the verbal operant conditioning experiment. J. of Personality soc. Psychol. *23:* 304–308 (1972).

Rosenthal, R.: Experimenter effects in behavioral research (Appleton Century Crofts, New York 1966).
Rogers, C. R.: On becoming a person (Houghton Mifflin, Boston 1961).
Rychlak, J. F.: A philosophy of science for personality theory (Houghton Mifflin, Boston 1968).
Rychlak, J. F.: A humanist looks at psychological science; in *Arnold and Cole* Nebraska symposium on motivation, vol. XXII (University of Nebraska Press, Lincoln 1975).
Skinner, B. F.: Beyond freedom and dignity (Knopf, New York 1971).

Cross-References

Abercrombie, M. L. J.: The anatomy of judgment: an investigation into the process of perception and reasoning (Hutchinson, London 1960).

Adler, A.: Problems of neurosis; (Harper & Row, New York 1964).

Adler, M. J.: Dialectic (Harcourt, Brace, New York 1927).

Adler, M. J.: The great ideas: a syntopicon; in *Hutchins* Great books of the western world, vol. 2, 3 (Encyclopedia Britannica, Chicago 1952).

Adorno, T. W.: Aufsätze zur Gesellschaftstheorie und Methodologie (Suhrkamp, Frankfurt 1970).

Ansbacher, H. L. and Ansbacher, R. R. (ed.): Superiority and social interest (Northwestern University Press, Evanston 1964).

Aristotle: Physics, and Topics; in *Hutchins* Great books of the western world, vol. 8, pp. 257–335, 143–223 (Encyclopedia Britannica, Chicago 1952).

Atkinson, J. W.: Motivational determinants of intellective performance and cumulative achievement; in *Atkinson and Raynor* Motivation and achievement, pp. 405–406 (Winston, Washington 1974).

Avant, L. L.: Psychophysics and scaling; in *Appley* Adaptation-level theory (Academic Press, New York 1971).

Bales, R. F.: Interaction process analysis (Addison Wesley, Cambridge 1951).

Bandura, A.: Principles of behavior modification (Holt, New York 1969).

Bannister, D.: Conceptual structure in thought-disordered schizophrenics. J. ment. Sci. *106:* 1230–1249 (1960).

Bannister, D.: The nature and measurement of schizophrenic thought disorder. J. ment. Sci. *108:* 325–342 (1962).

Bannister, D. and Fransella, F.: Inquiring man (Penguin, Baltimore 1971).

Bannister, D. and Salmon, P.: Schizophrenic thought disorder: specific or diffuse? Br. J. of med. Psychol. *39:* 215–219 (1966).

Bartlett, F. E.: Thinking: an experimental and social study (Basic Books, New York 1958).

Becker H. and Barnes, H. E.: Social thought from lore to science (Harren, Washington 1952).

Behar I. and Bevan, W.: The perceived duration of auditory and visual intervals. Cross-modal comparison and interaction. Am. J. Psychol. *74:* 17–26 (1961).

Bergler, E.: Laughter and the sense of humor (Intercontinental Medical Book, New York 1956).

Bergson, H.: Laughter: an essay on the meaning of comic (Macmillan, New York 1908).

Berlyne, D. E.: Aesthetics and psychobiology, pp. 43–99 (Appleton Century Crofts, New York 1971).

Berlyne, D. E.: Humor and its kin; in *Goldstein and McGhee* The psychology of humor (Academic Press, New York 1972).

Bettelheim, B.: Symbolic wounds; rev. ed. (Collier, New York 1962).

Bevan, W. and Pritchard, J. F.: Effects of 'subliminal' tones upon the judgment of loudness. J. exp. Psychol. *66:* 23–29 (1963).

Bickford, B. and Looft, W. R.: More on more: the mythology and actuality of children's understanding of relational terms. J. gen. Psychol. *123:* 139–143 (1973).

Bieri, J.: Cognitive complexity-simplicity and predictive hehavior. J. abnorm. soc. Psychol. *51:* 263–268 (1955).

Bieri, J.; Atkins, A. L.; Briar, S.; Leaman, R. L.; Miller, H., and Tripodi, T.: Clinical and social judgment (Wiley, New York 1966).

Bloom, B. S. (ed.): Taxonomy of educational objectives; in Handbook I. Cognitive domain (McKay, New York 1956).

Breuer, J. and Freud, S.: On the psychical mechanism of hysterical phenomena: preliminary communication; in *Strachey* The standard edition of the complete psychological works of Sigmund Freud, vol. II, pp. 1–17 (Hogarth, London 1955).

Brooks, C.: The community and the pariah; in *Vickery and Vickery* Light in August and the critical spectrum, pp. 168–183 (Wadsworth, Belmont 1971).

Bruyn, S. T.: The methodology of participant observation. Hum. Org. *22:* 224–235 (1963).

Bruyn, S. T.: The human perspective in sociology: the methodology of participant observation (Prentice Hall, Englewood Cliffs 1966).

Burtt, E. A.: The metaphysical foundations of modern physical science; rev. ed. (Doubleday, Garden City 1955).

Caligor, L. and May, R.: Dreams and symbols (Basic Books, New York 1968).

Chang, Kung-jang: The pulse-feeling of Chinese medicine. Ming Pao Mo. *6/9:* 41–44 (1971).

China Pictorial: vol. 2/284, pp. 13–14 (1970).

Chuang Tzu: Chuang Tzu; 2nd ed.; transl. by Giles (Kelly & Walsh, Shanghai 1926).

Clark, H. H.: Comprehending comparatives; in *Flores D'Arcais and Levelt* Advances in psycholinguistics, pp. 294–306 (North-Holland, Amsterdam 1970).

Cofer, C. N.: Constructive processes in memory. Am. Sci. *61:* 537–543 (1973).

Comte, A.: Lettres d'Auguste Comte à divers, vol. I (Fonds Typographique, Paris 1902).

Coombs, C. H.: A theory of data (Wiley, New York 1964).

Cooper, L.: An Aristotelian theory of comedy (Harcourt, New York 1922).

Cronbach, L. J.: Beyond the two disciplines of scientific psychology. Am. Psychol. *30:* 116–127 (1975).

Datan, N.: To be a woman in Israel. Sch. Rev. *80:* 319–332 (1972).

Datan, N.: Your daughters shall prophesy: ancient and contemporary perspectives on the women of Israel; in *Curtis and Chertoff* Israel: social structure and change (Transaction Books, New Brunswick 1973).

Datan, N.: Astarte, Moses, and Mary: perspectives on the sexual dialectic in Canaanite, Judaic, and Christian tradition; in *Riegel and Meacham* The developing individual in a changing world, vol. 1 (Mouton, The Hague 1975).

Datan, N.: Ecological antecedents and sex role consequences in traditional and modern Israeli sub-cultures; in *Schlegel* Emergent women (University of Pittsburgh Press, Pittsburgh in press).

Deese, J.: Psychology as science and art (Harcourt, Brace, & Jovanovich, New York 1972).

Denis-Prinzhorn, M.: Perceptions des distances et constance des grandeurs. Etude génétique. Arch. Psychol., Genève *37:* 181–309 (1960).

Dessoir, M.: Ästhetik und allgemeine Kunstwissenschaft (Enke, Stuttgart 1923).

Devereux, G.: From anxiety to method in behavioral research (Mouton, The Hague 1967).

Dewey, J. and Bentley, A. F.: Knowing and the known (Beacon, Boston 1954).

Dexter, L. A.: Elite and specialized interviewing (Northwestern University Press, Evanston 1970).

Dinnerstein, D.; Michel, G., and Byrwa, D.: Inter- and intramural context effects on kinesthetically perceived breadth (unpublished, Rutgers University, New Brunswick 1968).

Donaldson, M. and Balfour, G.: Less is more: a study of language comprehension in children. Br. J. Psychol. *59:* 461–471 (1968).

Duck, S. W.: Personal relationships and personal constructs (Wiley, New York 1973).

Dulany, D. E.: The place of hypotheses and intentions: an analysis of verbal control in verbal conditioning; in *Eriksen* Behavior and awareness: a symposium of research and interpretation, pp. 102–129 (Duke University Press, Durham 1962).

Eastman, M.: The sense of humor (Scribners, New York 1921).

Ellul, J.: The technological society (Vintage, New York 1964).

Erikson, E. H.: Childhood and society; rev. ed. (Norton, New York 1963).

Fang, Thomè H.: The Chinese view of life (Union Press, Hong Kong 1957).

Faulkner, W.: Light in August (Modern Library, New York 1959).

Fenichel, O.: Über die Psychoanalyse als Keim einer zukünftigen dialektisch-materialistischen Psychologie; in Marxismus, Psychoanalyse, Sexpol 1, pp. 229–249 (Fischer, Frankfurt 1970).

Feuer, L. S.: Einstein and the generations of science (Basic Books, New York 1974).

Fiebleman, J. K.: In praise of comedy (Macmillan, New York 1939).

Findlay, J. N.: The philosophy of Hegel: an introduction and re-examination (Collier, New York 1958).

Flavell, J. H.: Cognitive changes in adulthood; in *Goulet and Baltes* Life-span developmental psychology: research and theory, pp. 247–253 (Academic Press, New York 1970).

Flavell, J. H. and Wohlwill, J. F.: Formal and functional aspects of cognitive development; in *Elkind and Flavell* Studies in cognitive development, pp. 67–120 (Oxford University Press, New York 1969).

Freud, S.: Der Witz und seine Beziehung zum Unbewussten (Leipzig and Vienna 1905).

Freud, S.: New introductory lectures on psychoanalysis (Norton, New York 1933).

Freud, S.: The interpretation of dreams; in *Strachey* The standard edition of the complete psychological works of Sigmund Freud, vol. IV, V (Hogarth, London 1953).

Freud, S.: Fragment of an analysis of a case of hysteria; in *Strachey* The standard edition of the complete psychological works of Sigmund Freud, vol. VII, pp. 3–112 (Hogarth, London 1953).

Freud, S.: The origins of psycho-analysis: Letters to Wilhelm Fliess, drafts and notes: 1887–1902; in *Bonaparte, Freud and Kris;* authorized translation by Mosbacher and Strachey (Basic Books, New York 1954).

Freud, S.: On narcissism: an introduction; in *Strachey* The standard edition of the complete psychological works of Sigmund Freud, vol. XIV, pp. 67–102 (Hogarth, London 1957).

Freud, S.: The antithetical meaning of primal words; in *Strachey* The standard edition of the complete psychological works of Sigmund Freud, vol. XI, pp. 153–162 (Hogarth, London 1957).

Freud, S.: Psycho-analytic notes on an autobiographical account of a case of paranoia; in *Strachey* The standard edition of the complete psychological works of Sigmund Freud, vol XII, pp. 1–82 (Hogarth, London 1958).

Freud, S.: Civilization and its discontents (Norton, New York 1961).

Freud, S.: The ego and the id, and other works; in ***Strachey*** The standard edition of the complete psychological works of Sigmund Freud, vol. XIX (Hogarth, London 1961).

Freud, S.: The future of an illusion; in ***Strachey*** The standard edition of the complete psychological works of Sigmund Freud, pp. 1–56 (Hogarth, London 1961).

Freud, S.: The neuro-psychoses of defence; in ***Strachey*** The standard edition of the complete psychological works of Sigmund Freud, vol. III, pp. 45–61 (Hogarth, London 1962).

Freud, S.: Introductory lectures on psycho-analysis. Part III; in ***Strachey*** The standard edition of the complete psychological works of Sigmund Freud, vol. XVI (Hogarth, London 1963).

Freud, S.: A case of successful treatment by hypnotism; in ***Strachey*** The standard edition of the complete psychological works of Sigmund Freud, vol. I, pp. 115–128 (Hogarth, London 1966).

Freud, S.: Project for a scientific psychology; in ***Strachey*** The standard edition of the complete psychological works of Sigmund Freud, vol. I, pp. 281–397 (Hogarth, London 1966).

Friedman, N.: The social nature of psychological research (Basic Books, New York 1967).

From, F.: Perception of other people (Columbia University Press, New York 1971).

Fung, Yu-lan: A history of Chinese philosophy, vol. 1; transl. by Bodde (Princeton University Press, Princeton 1952).

Furth, H. G.: Piaget, IQ, and the nature-nurture controversy. Hum. Dev. *16:* 61–73 (1973).

Galtung, J.: Theory and methods of social research. Oslo: Universitetsforlaget, 1967.

Giorgi, A.: Psychology as a human science (Harper & Row, New York 1970).

Glidewell, J. C.: The entry problem in consultation. J. soc. Issues *15:* 51–60 (1959).

Goethe, J. W.: Maximen und Reflexionen (Verlag der Goethe-Gesellschaft, Weimar 1907).

Gouldner, A. W.: The norm of reciprocity. Am. sociol. Rev. *25:* 161–179 (1960).

Gregory, J. C.: The nature of laughter (Kegan, London 1924).

Grieg, J. Y. T.: The psychology of laughter and comedy (Dodd, Mead, New York 1923).

Griffith, R.: Anthropodology: man a-foot; in *von Bayer and Griffith* Conditio humana, pp. 84–102 (Springer, New York 1966).

Griffiths, J. A.; Shantz, C. A., and Sigel, I. E.: A methodological problem in conservation studies: the use of relational terms. Child Dev. *38:* 841–848 (1967).

Gutmann, D.: An exploration of ego configurations in middle and later life; in ***Neugarten et al.*** Personality in middle and late life (Atherton Press, New York 1964).

Gutmann, D.: Men, women, and the parental imperative. Commentary. December 1973.

Gutmann, D.: Parenthood: key to the comparative study of the life cycle; in ***Datan and Ginsberg*** Life-span developmental psychology: normative life crises (Academic Press, New York 1975).

Habermas, J.: Knowledge and human interests (Beacon, Boston 1971).

Haldane, J. B. S.: The Marxist philosophy and the sciences (Allen & Unwin, London 1938).

Hauser, A.: The social history of art. Vol. I, Prehistoric, ancient-Oriental, Greece and Rome, middle ages; vol. II, Renaissance, mannerism, baroque; vol. III, Rococo, classicism, romanticism; vol. IV, Naturalism, impressionism, the film age (Vintage, New York 1951).

Hayworth, D.: The social origins and functions of laughter. Psychol. Rev. *35:* 367–384 (1928).

Hegel, G. W. F.: The philosophy of history, and The philosophy of right; in ***Hutchins*** Great books of the western world, vol. 46, pp. 153–369, 1–150 (Encyclopedia Britannica, Chicago 1952).

Hegel, G. W. F.: Phänomenologie des Geistes (Suhrkamp, Frankfurt 1969); The phenomenology of mind (Harper-Torch Books, New York 1967).

Hegel, G. W. F.: Wissenschaft der Logik (Suhrkamp, Frankfurt 1969); Science of logic (Allen & Unwin, London 1929).

Heidegger, M.: The origin of the work of art; in *Hofstader and Kuhns* Philosophies of art and beauty; pp. 649–701 (Modern Library and Random House, New York 1964).

Helson, H.: Adaptation level theory (Harper & Row, New York 1964).

Hobbes, T.: Leviathan; in *Hutchins* Great books of the western world, vol. 23, pp. 49–283 (Encyclopedia Britannica, Chicago 1952).

Hogan, R.: Moral conduct and moral character: a psychological perspective. Psychol. Bull. *79:* 217–232 (1973).

Hook, S.: From Hegel to Marx (University of Michigan Press, Ann Arbor 1962).

Hooper, F. H.: Cognitive assessment across the lifespan: methodological implication of the organismic approach; in *Nesselroade and Reese* Life-span developmental psychology: methodological issues, pp. 299–316 (Academic Press, New York 1972).

Hovland, C. I.; Harvey, O. J., and Sherif, M,: Assimilation and contrast effects in reactions to communication and attitude change. J. abnorm. soc. Psychol. *55:* 244–252 (1957).

Hsu, F. L. K.: American and Chinese: two ways of life (Schuman, New York 1953).

Hughes, E. C.: Introduction; in *Junker* An introduction to the social sciences, pp. iii–xiii (University of Chicago Press, Chicago 1960).

Hui-neng: Sūtra spoken by the sixth patriarch on the high seat of 'the treasure of the law' (in Chinese), preface dated 1290 (Buddhist Book Distributor, Hong Kong 1929).

Husserl, E.: Die Krisis der europäischen Wissenschaften und die transzendentale Phänomenologie (Nijhoff, Haag 1962).

Huttenlocher, J. and Higgins, E. T.: Adjectives, comparatives, and syllogism. Psychol. Rev. *78:* 487–504 (1971).

I Ching (in Chinese); in *Sung* The text of Yi King and its appendices: a Chinese original with English translations (The China Modern Education, Shanghai 1935).

Inhelder, B. and Piaget, J.: The early growth of logic in the child (Norton, New York, 1969).

Janet, P.: The major symptoms of hysteria; 2nd ed. (Macmillan, New York 1920).

Jaspars, J. M. F.: On social perception (Lectura, Leiden 1966).

Jay, M.: The dialectical imagination (Little, Brown, Boston 1973).

Johnson, P. J. and White, R. M.: Concept of dimensionality and reversal shift performance in children. J. exp. Child Psychol. *5:* 223–227 (1957).

Jones, E.: The life and work of Sigmund Freud: the last phase, vol. 3 (Basic Books, New York 1957).

Jung, C. G.: Psychology and literature; in modern man in search of a soul; transl. by *Dell and Baynes*, pp. 152–173 (Harcourt, Brace & World, New York 1933).

Jung, C. G.: The practice of psychotherapy; in *Read, Fordham and Adler* The collected works of C. G. Jung, vol. 16. Bollingen Series XX.16 (Pantheon Books / Routledge & Kegan, New York/London 1954).

Jung, C. G.: The development of personality; in *Read, Fordham and Adler* The collected works of C. G. Jung, vol. 17. Bollingen Series XX.17 (Pantheon Books, New York 1961).

Kagan, J.: On the need for relativism. Am. Psychol. *22:* 131–142 (1967).

Kant, I.: The critique of pure reason; in *Hutchins* Great books of the western world, vol. 42, pp. 1–250 (Encyclopedia Britannica, Chicago 1952).

Keith-Spiegel, P.: Early conceptions of humor: varieties and issues; in *Goldstein and McGhee* The psychology of humor, pp. 4–34 (Academic Press, New York 1972).

Kelly, G. A.: The psychology of personal constructs (Norton, New York 1955).

Kendler, H. H. and Kendler, T. S.: Vertical and horizontal processes in problem solving. Psychol. Rev. *69:* 1–16 (1962).

Kendler, H. H. and Kendler, T. S.: Reversal-shift behavior: some basic issues. Psychol. Bull. *72:* 229–232 (1969).

Knox, I.: Towards a philosophy of humor. J. Phil. *48:* 541–548 (1951).

Koestler, A.: The act of creation (Hutchinson, London 1964).

Koffka, K.: Principles of gestalt psychology (Harcourt, Brace, New York 1935).

Kohler, W.: The mentality of apes; transl. by Winters (Routledge & Kagan, London 1925).

Kominski, C. A. and Coppinger, N. W.: The Müller-Lyer illusion and Piaget's test for the development of the conservation of space in a group of older institutionalized veterans (William and Mary College, Williamsburg 1968).

Koplon, D.: Dichotomy in cognition and reversal and non-reversal shifting; unpublished diss. State University of New York, Albany (1970).

Kosik, K.: Dialektik des Konkreten (Suhrkamp, Frankfurt 1971).

Kuenne, M. R.: Experimental investigation of the relation of language to transposition behavior in young children. J. exp. Psychol. *36:* 471–490 (1946).

Kuhn, T. S.: The structure of scientific revolutions; 2nd ed. (University of Chicago Press, Chicago 1970).

Kuo, You-yuh: Psychology in Communist China. Psychol. Rec. *21:* 95–105 (1971).

Kuo, You-yuh: Family constellation in the Chinese languages. J. indiv. Psychol. *27:* 181–184 (1971).

Kvale, S.: The technological paradigm of psychological research. J. phenomenol. Psychol. *3:* 143–159 (1973).

Kvale, S.: Memory and dialectics: some reflections on Ebbinghaus and Mao Tse-tung. Hum. Dev. *18* (in press, 1975).

Kvale, S.: Meanings as data and human technology (unpublished, University of Aarhus, 1975).

Kvale, S. and Grenness, C. E.: Skinner and Sartre: towards a radical phenomenology of behavior? Rev. existent. Psychol. Psychiat. *7:* 128–150 (1967).

Landfield, A. W.: Personal construct systems in psychotherapy (Rand McNally, Chicago 1971).

Langer, S. K.: Philosophy in a new key (Penguin Books, New York 1948).

Laurendeau, M. and Pinard, A.: The development of the concept of space in the child (International Universities Press, New York 1970).

Levy, L. H. and Dugan, R. D.: A factorial study of personal constructs. J. consult. Psychol. *20:* 53–57 (1956).

Lewin, K.: Behavior and development as a function of total situation; in *Carmichael* Manual of child psychology; 4th ed. pp. 918–970 (Wiley, New York 1954).

Lin Yutang: The wisdom of Lao Tze (Modern Library, New York 1948).

Locke, J.: An essay concerning human understanding; in *Hutchins* Great books of the western world, vol. 35, pp. 85–395 (Encyclopedia Britannica, Chicago 1952).

Lourenço, S. V.: Social conflict resolution and the dialectic; unpublished diss. University of Chicago, Chicago (1974).

Ludovici, A. M.: The secret of laughter (Constable, London 1932).

Lukacs, G.: History and class consciousness (Merlin, London 1971).

Lynch, W.: Images of hope (New American Library, New York 1965).

Magill, F. N. and McGreal, I. P.: Masterpieces of world philosophy, vol. I, II, (Salem Press, New York 1961).

Maier, N. R. F.: A gestalt theory of humor. Br. J. Psychol. *23:* 69–74 (1932).

Mancuso, J. C. (ed.): Readings for a cognitive theory of personality (Holt, Rinehart, & Winston, New York 1970).

Mandler, G. and Kessen, W.: The language of psychology (Wiley, New York 1964).

Mao, Tse-tung: On practice (1937); in Selected works of Mao Tse-tung, vol. I, pp. 295–310 (Foreign Languages Press, Peking 1967).

Mao, Tse-tung: On contradiction (1937); in Selected works of Mao Tse-tung, vol. I, pp. 311–347 (Foreign Languages Press, Peking 1967).

Mao, Tse-tung: Four essays on philosophy (Foreign Languages Press, Peking 1968).

Marx, K.: Capital; in *Hutchins* Great books of the western world, vol. 50, pp. 1–393 (Encyclopedia Britannica, Chicago 1952).

May, R.: Power and innocence (Norton, New York 1971).

McCain, G. and Segal, E. M.: The game of science (Brooks / Cole, Belmont 1969).

McComas, H. C.: The origin of laughter. Psychol. Rev. *30:* 45–55 (1923).

McDougall, W.: The theory of laughter. Nature, Lond. *67:* 318–319 (1903).

McGhee, P.: On the cognitive origins of incongruity humor: fantasy assimilation versus reality assimilation; in *Goldstein and McGhee* The psychology of humor, pp. 61–79 (Academic Press, New York 1972).

McGuire, W. (ed.): The Freud / Jung letters: the correspondence between Sigmund Freud and C. G. Jung (Princeton University Press, Princeton 1974).

McLaughlin, G. H.: Psychologic: a possible alternative to Piaget's formulation. Br. J. educ. Psychol. *33:* 61–67 (1963).

Mead, G. H.: Mind, self, and society (University of Chicago Press, Chicago 1934).

Mead, M.: Male and female (Morrow, New York 1949).

Menon, V. K.: A theory of laughter (Allen & Unwin, London 1931).

Merleau-Ponty, M.: Phenomenology of perception (Routledge & Kegan / Humanities Press, London / New York 1962).

Miller, S. A.: Contradiction, surprise, and cognitive change: the effects of disconfirmation of belief on conservers and nonconservers; unpublished University of Michigan, Ann Arbor (1972).

Moore, C. A.: The Chinese mind (East-West Center Press, Honolulu 1967).

Moore, C. A.: The Indian mind (East-West Center Press, Honolulu 1967).

Muller-Vollmer, K.: Towards a phenomenological theory of literature (Mouton, The Hague 1963).

Murphy, R. E.: The dialectic of social life: alarms and excursions in anthropological theory (Basic Books, New York 1971).

Nākāmura, H.: Ways of thinking of eastern peoples: India-China-Tibet-Japan (East-West Center Press, Honolulu 1964).

Needham, J.: Science and civilization in China, vol. I (University Press, Cambridge 1953).

Neisser, U.: Cognitive psychology (Appleton Century Crofts, New York 1967; quotations by permission of Prentice-Hall, Englewood Cliffs).

Neugarten, B. L.: The awareness of middle age; in *Neugarten* Middle age and aging (University of Chicago Press, Chicago 1968).

Neugarten, B. L. and Gutmann, D.: Age-sex roles and personality in middle age: a thematic apperception study. Psychol. Monogr. *72:* No. 17, whole No. 470 (1958).

Neugarten, B. L. and Moore, J. W.: The changing age-status system; in *Neugarten* Middle age and aging (The University of Chicago Press, Chicago 1968).

Ong, W.: The presence of the word (Simon & Schuster, New York 1967).

Orne, M. T.: On the social psychology of the psychological experiment: with particular reference to demand characteristics and their implications. Am. Psychol. *17:* 776–783 (1962).

Osgood, C. E. and Richards, M. M.: From yang and yin to and or but. Language *49:* 380–412 (1973).

Osgood, C. E.; Suci, G. J., and Tannenbaum, P. H.: The measurement of meaning (University of Illinois Press, Urbana 1957).

Page, M. M.: Demand characteristics and the verbal operant conditioning experiment. J. Personality soc. Psychol. *23:* 304–308 (1972).

Paivio, A.: Language and knowledge of the world. Educ. Researcher *3:* 5–12 (1974).

Paolucci, A. and Paolucci, H.: Hegel: on tragedy (Doubleday, Garden City 1962).

Papalia, D. E.: The status of several conservation abilities across the life span. Hum. Dev. *15:* 229–243 (1972).

Parducci, A.; Calfee, R. C.; Marshall, L. M., and Davidson, L. P.: Context effects in judgment: adaptation level as a function of mean, midpoint, and median of the stimuli. J. exp. psychol. *60:* 65–77 (1960).

Parducci, A. and Marshall, L. M.: Context effects in the judgments of length. Am. J. Psychol. *74:* 576–583 (1961).

Pepper, S. C.: World hypotheses (University of California Press, Berkeley 1942).

Piaget, J.: Play, dreams, and imitation in childhood (Norton, New York 1962).

Piaget, J.: The origin of intelligence in children (Norton, New York 1963).

Piaget, J.: The moral judgment of the child (Free Press, Glencoe 1965).

Piaget, J.: The child's conception of number (Norton, New York 1965).

Piaget, J.: Intellectual evolution from adolescence to adulthood. Hum. Dev. *15:* 1–12 (1972).

Piaget, J. and Inhelder, B.: The child's conception of space (Routledge & Kegan, London 1956; in paperback: Norton, New York 1967).

Piaget, J.; Inhelder, B., and Szeminska, A.: The child's conception of geometry (Harper Torchbooks, New York 1964).

Plato: Cratylus, Parmenides, Philebus, Sophist, Statesman, and Symposium; in *Hutchins* Great books of the western world, vol. 7, pp 85–639 (Encyclopedia Britannica, Chicago 1952).

Plessner, H.: Laughing and crying: a study of the limits of behavior (Northwestern University Press, Evanston 1970).

Pribram, K.: Conflicting patterns of thought (Public Affairs Press, Washington 1949).

Rank, O.: Will therapy and truth and reality (Knopf, New York 1945).

Reich, W.: Dialektischer Materialismus und Psychoanalyse. Unter dem Banner des Marxismus (1929).

Ricoeur, P.: The symbolism of evil; transl. by Buchanan (Harper & Row, New York 1967).

Rieff, P.: Freud: the mind of the moralist (Anchor, New York 1959).

Riegel, K. F.: On the history of psychological gerontology; in *Eisdorfer and Lawton* The psychology of adult development and aging, pp. 37–68 (American Psychological Association, Washington 1973).

Riegel, K. F.: Development, drop and death. Devl. Psychol. *6:* 306–319 (1972).

Riegel, K. F.: Developmental psychology and society: some historical and ethical considerations; in *Nesselroade and Reese* Life-span developmental psychology: methodological issues pp. 1–23 (Academic Press, New York 1972).

Riegel, K. F.: The influence of economic and political ideologies upon the development of psychology. Psychol. Bull. *78:* 129–141 (1972).

Riegel, K. F.: Time and change in the development of the individual and society; in *Reese* Advances in child development and behavior, vol. 7, pp. 81–113 (Academic Press, New York 1972).

Riegel, K. F.: All the trouble with linguistics. Int. J. Psycholinguist. (in press, 1975).

Riegel, K. F.: Introduction to developmental and historical structuralism; in *Riegel* and *Rosenwald*, Structure and transformation: developmental and historical aspects, pp. 36–57 (Wiley, New York 1975).

Rogers, C. R.: On becoming a person (Houghton Mifflin, Boston 1961).

Rosenthal, R.: Experimenter effects in behavioral research (Appleton Century Crofts, New York 1966).

Royce, J. R.: Psychology at the crossroads; in *Royce* Psychology and the symbol, pp. 3–25 (Random House, New York 1965).

Rubinsteijn, S. L.: Prinzipien und Wege der Entwicklung der Psychologie. (Akademie-Verlag, Berlin 1963).

Russell, B.: An inquiry into meaning and truth (Penguin, Harmondsworth 1962).

Rychlak, J. F.: A philosophy of science for personality theory (Houghton Mifflin, Boston 1968).

Rychlak, J. F.: Introduction to personality and psychotherapy: a theory-construction approach (Houghton Mifflin, Boston 1973).

Rychlak, J. F.: A humanist looks at psychological science; in *Arnold and Cole* Nebraska symposium on motivation, vol. XXII (University of Nebraska Press, Lincoln 1975).

Samelson, F.: History, origin, myth and ideology: 'discovery' of social psychology. J. Theory soc. Behav. *4:* 217–231 (1974).

Sanders, S.; Laurendeau, M., and Bergeron, J.: Aging and the concept of space: the conservation of surface. J. Geront. *21:* 281–285 (1966).

Sandler, G. B.: Improving participant observation: the T-group as an answer. J. appl. behav. Sci. *9:* 31–61 (1973).

Sarbin, T. R.; Taft, R. and Bailey, D. E.: Clinical inference and cognitive theory (Holt, Rinehart, & Winston, New York 1960).

Sartre, J.-P.: The problem of method (Methuen, London 1963).

Schopenhauer, A.: Die Welt als Wille und Vorstellung (Brockhaus, Leipzig 1819).

Scott, W. A.: Structure of natural cognitions. J. Personality soc. Psychol. *12:* 261–268 (1969).

Sherif, M. and Hovland, C. I.: Social judgment: assimilation and contrast effects in communication and attitude change (Yale University Press, New Haven 1961).

Sherif, C.; Sherif M., and Nebergall, R. E.: Attitude and attitude change: the social judgment – involvement approach (Saunders, Philadelphia 1965).

Sherif, M.; Taub, D., and Hovland, C. I.: Assimilation and contrast effects of anchoring stimuli on judgments. J. exp. Psychol. *55:* 150–155 (1958).

Sidis, B.: The psychology of laughter (Appleton, New York 1913).

Skinner, B. F.: Cumulative record (Appleton Century Crofts, New York 1961).

Skinner, B. F.: Beyond freedom and dignity (Knopf, New York 1971).

Skinner, B. F.: About behaviorism (Knopf, New York 1974).

Skjervheim, H.: Objectivism and the study of man (Universitetsforlaget, Oslo 1959).

Smedslund, J.: Meanings, implications and universals: towards a psychology of man. Scand. J. Psychol. *10:* 1–15 (1969).

Spence, K. W.: Behavior theory and conditioning (Yale University Press, New Haven 1956).

Spencer, H.: The physiology of laughter. Macmillan's Mag. *1:* 395–402 (1860).

Stace, W. T.: The philosophy of Hegel (Dover, New York 1955).

Stanley, H. M.: Remarks on tickling and laughing. Am. J. Psychol. *9:* 235–240 (1898).

Strasser, S.: Phenomenology and the human sciences (Duquesne University Press, Pittsburgh 1963).

Sully, J.: Essay on laughter (Longmans, Green, New York 1902).

Suzuki, D. T.: The essentials of Zen Buddhism; in *Phillips* (Dutton, New York 1962).

Tao Te Ching (in Chinese) (Hsuan-Feng, Taipei 1950).

Terman, L. M. and Merrill, M. A.: Stanford-Binet Intelligence Scale (Houghton Mifflin, Boston 1960).

Thurstone, L. L. and Chave, E. J.: The measurement of attitude (University of Chicago Press, Chicago 1929).

Toffler, A.: Future shock (Random House, New York 1961).

Trilling, L.: Sincerity and authenticity (Harvard University Press, Cambridge 1972).

Turbayne, C.: The myth of metaphor (University of South Carolina Press, Columbia 1970).

Van den Daele, L. D.: Qualitative models in developmental analysis. Devl. Psychol. *1:* 303–310 (1969).

Vansina, L. S.: Aspects psychologiqiues de la fonction de conseil. Ned. Tijdschr. Psychol. *25:* 3 (1970).

Verhoven, N.: The philosophy of wonder (Macmillan, New York 1972).

Vygotsky, L. S.: The psychology of art (MIT Press, Cambridge 1971).

Wallis, W. O.: 'Why do we laugh? ' Scient. Mon. *15:* 343–347 (1922).

Watson, J. B.: Psychology as a natural science. The failure of psychology as a mental science; in *Skinner* Readings in psychology, pp. 809–811 (Holt, Rinehart & Winston, New York 1935).

Webb, E. J.; Campbell, D. J.; Schwartz, R. D.; and Sechrest, L.: Unobtrusive measures in the social sciences (Rand McNally, Chicago 1966).

Weber, J. P.: The psychology of art (Delta Books, New York 1969).

Werner, H.: Einführung in die Entwicklungspsychologie (Barth, Leipzig 1926). Comparative psychology of mental development (Follett, New York 1948).

White, B.: The initial coordination of sensorimotor schemas in human infants – Piaget's ideas of the role of experience; in *Elkind and Flavell* Studies in cognitive development (Oxford University Press, New York 1969).

White, R. M. and Johnson, P. J.: Concept of dimensionality and optional shift performance in nursery school children. J. exp. Child Psychol. *6:* 113–119 (1968).

Whyte, W. F.: Street corner society; 2nd ed. (University of Chicago Press, Chicago 1955).

Wimsatt, W. K.: The structure of the 'concrete universal' in literature; in *Schorer, Miles and McKenzie* Criticism, pp. 393–407 (Harcourt, Brace & World, New York 1958).

Winterstein, A.: Contributions to the problem of humor. Psychoanal. Q. *3:* 303–316 (1934).

Wozniak, R. H.: Dialecticism and structuralism in Soviet philosophy and psychology; in *Riegel and Rosenwald* Structure and transformation: developmental and historical aspects, pp. 176–192 (Wiley, New York 1975).

Subject Index

Name Index